Recent Results in Cancer Research 72

Fortschritte der Krebsforschung
Progrès dans les recherches sur le cancer

Cawley Burns Hayhoe

Hairy-Cell Leukaemia

With 64 Figures and 4 Tables

Springer-Verlag
Berlin Heidelberg New York 1980

Dr. John C. Cawley

University College Hospital, Department of Haematology, Gower Street, GB – London WC1E 6AU

Dr. Gordon F. Burns

Clinical Research Unit, Walter and Eliza Hall Institute of Medical Research, Royal Melbourne Hospital, AUS – Melbourne, Victoria

Professor Frank G. J. Hayhoe

Department of Haematological Medicine, School of Clinical Medicine, University of Cambridge, Hills Road, GB – Cambridge CB2 2QL

Sponsored by the Swiss League against Cancer

ISBN-13:978-3-642-81439-6 e-ISBN-13:978-3-642-81437-2
DOI: 10.1007/978-3-642-81437-2

Library of Congress Cataloging in Publication Data. Main entry under title: Hairy-cell leukaemia. (Recent results in cancer research; 72) „Sponsored by the Swiss League against Cancer." Bibliography: p. Includes index. 1. Leukaemia, Hairy cell. I. Cawley, J. C. II. Burns, G. F., 1947– III. Hayhoe, F. G. J. IV. Schweizerische Nationalliga für Krebsbekämpfung und Krebsforschung. V. Series. [DNLM: 1. Leukaemia, Hairy cell. W1 RE106P v. 72/WH250 H153] RC261.R35 vol. 72 [RC643] 616.99'4s [616.99'419] 80-11719

Softcover reprint of the hardcover 1st edition 1980

2125/3140–543210

Acknowledgements

We are indebted to many physicians, including Drs. F. K. Amroliwalla, A. J. Child, T. J. Deeble, A. P. Dick, M. Edwards, J. Gobert-Jones, A. H. Goldstone, K. Hunt, G. N. W. Kerrigan, M. King, C. G. L. Raper, J. K. H. Rees and R. Sibbald, who enabled us to study their cases of HCL.
We should like to thank various other colleagues, including Prof. C. C. Bird and Drs. C. R. Barker, I. Barrett, A. Bevan, J. Gooi, J. L. Smith, H. Williams, M. Zuzel, and J. Binns, R. J. Flemans and C. P. Worman, for help and collaboration with certain aspects of the work presented in this book.
Invaluable secretarial assistance was given by Miss H. Collingwood, Miss J. Thomson and Miss K. Woolley.
Special acknowledgement is due to Prof. G. P. McNicol and Dr. B.E. Roberts, who assisted JCC in every possible way during the completion of this work.

Contents

1 Introduction

Hairy-cell leukaemia (HCL) is an established clinicopathological entity typified by a chronic picture of substantial splenomegaly, less frequent hepatomegaly, and only inconspicuous lymphadenopathy. Central to the diagnosis is the pathognomonic hairy cell (HC), a distinctive mononuclear cell that circulates in varying numbers and infiltrates a variety of organs, including the bone marrow and spleen. Peripheral pancytopenia is often present, and circulating HCs may be infrequent. HCs are invariably present in the bone marrow; but, perhaps because of the extensive fibrosis characteristic of the disease, the marrow is frequently difficult to aspirate, and confirmation of the diagnosis may require histopathological examination of biopsy material.

The incidence of the disease has been given as 2% of leukaemias [29, 319] or as approximately 1% of identifiable lymphomas [230]. Our own experience of collecting cases in the United Kingdom leads us to expect that at any given time one patient with HCL will be attending a clinic serving some 150,000 people.

The first complete description of what is now understood as HCL was given by ROSENTHAL and LEE in 1951 [319]. Other reports of the same entity followed [157], but it was the detailed report from BOURONCLE et al. in 1958 [29] that led to the disease being widely regarded as a distinct entity. These authors clearly identified "reticulum cells" with a serrated border in a group of 26 patients presenting a well-defined clinicopathological picture. Subsequent work has amply confirmed the existence of HCL as a distinct clinicopathological entity [40, 70, 202, 226, 386].

BOURONCLE's group chose to call this distinct entity leukaemic reticuloendotheliosis, and in recent years the terms hairy-cell leukaemia [298, 337] and leukaemic reticuloendotheliosis have come to be regarded by many authors as synonymous. Originally, however, leukaemic reticuloendotheliosis had a broader usage, covering a group of conditions now regarded as several different diseases. Thus, the term leukämische Reticuloendotheliose was first introduced by EWALD in 1923 [116] to describe a form of monocytic leukaemia [18, 200]. Later, the term was applied to monocytic leukaemias of both pure (SCHILLING) and mixed (NAEGELI) types [18, 110, 123, 157, 200] and also to lymphoid disorders, including a variety of non-Hodgkin's lymphomas [123, 157, 228]. This rather broad use of the term leukaemic reticuloendotheliosis may account, at least in part, for the large number of confusing terms that have been regarded as synonyms for the entity [29] but have probably often not referred to HCL. These include histiocytic leukaemia, malignant leukaemic reticulohistiocytosis, histioleukaemia, reticulosis, malignant reticulosis, and aleukaemic reticulosis (early literature reviewed by BOURONCLE et al. [29]). More recent terms clearly referring to HCL are histiolymphocytose médullaire et splénique [26, 124], reticulum cell leukaemia [226], chronic reticulolymphocytic leukaemia [325], and lymphoid myelofibrosis [111, 209]. In addition, there are the various translations of hairy-cell leukaemia, which include leucémie à tricholeucocytes and Haarzell-Leukämie.

In recent years HCL has increasingly become the preferred name [335, 337]. Certainly, while there continues to be controversy about the nature and origin of the pathognomonic cells of the disease, this descriptive term has the advantage of not carrying possibly incorrect connotations regarding the nature and origin of the abnormal cells, while leaving no room for doubt about the clinicopathological entity under consideration [337]. In this monograph, therefore, we propose to use the term hairy-cell leukaemia, or HCL, throughout, concurring with SYMMERS statement [366] that 'It is difficult to conceive how a disease that has become so widely known as "hairy cell leukaemia" can ever be referred to by any more mundane name'.

Although the disease has now been clearly recognized for more than 20 years, HCL remains the subject of much attention and controversy. There are many reasons for the continuing high level of interest in the disease. The distinctive clinicopathological picture, with its bizarre pathognomonic HCs, would guarantee the interest of all morphological haematologists even without the numerous remaining clinical problems associated with HCL. For example, difficulty may be encountered with the diagnosis [117, 202, 239], and HCL may still be mistaken for acute lymphocytic or undifferentiated leukaemia, for a variety of malignant lymphomas with bone-marrow and blood involvement, or even for chronic lymphocytic leukaemia or myelofibrosis [29, 40, 63, 70, 201, 202, 204, 239, 258, 284, 339, 387]. Such misdiagnoses may have severe consequences, since vigorous chemotherapy is usually contraindicated in HCL (see Chap. 2 and review by CATOVSKY [63]). Furthermore, the lack of regularly effective treatment for the more rapidly progressive or end stages of the disease remains a therapeutic challenge [239]. A number of other problems continue to provide subjects for more clinically oriented investigation. Among these are: the role of splenectomy [29, 40, 63, 70, 189, 202, 298, 386]; the nature of the spontaneous remissions occasionally observed [28, 226]; and the recognition of abnormalities in apparently unrelated cell types (e.g., abnormalities of platelet function [151, 202, 231]).

The HC itself has proved a major stimulus of study by both haematologists and immunologists. There is still controversy about the precise nature of the HC, since this cell has features in common with both B lymphocytes and monocytes; indeed, a recent report from the World Health Organization and the International Union of Immunological Societies described HCL as unclassified in type [19]. The early literature considered the HC to be derived from primitive undifferentiated reticulum cells whose normal progeny would have included cells of the lymphoid, myeloid, and monocyte-macrophage series [29, 258]. The hybrid features of HCs are readily understood in terms of this scheme; but since more recent work has shown that the lymphoid and monocytoid series develop independently from a very early stage, the existence of such a hybrid cell type has proved both intriguing and perplexing.

Not only do HCs possess hybrid lymphoid-monocytoid features, but they also possess several features that are distinctive [51, 63, 177, 202, 387]. This has led to continued interest in the possibility that hairy cells are not directly related to either B-lymphoid or monocytoid cells, but rather derived from a normal, still undefined counterpart [51, 93, 182, 361]. The purpose of this monograph is to present our personal clinical and laboratory experience of 30 cases of HCL and to relate this to the existing literature on the subject. This work is intended to provide an assessment of the present state of knowledge of HCL and to clarify or resolve some of the controversial issues raised above. At the same time, however, it is acknowledged that many aspects of HCL remain perplexing, and it is hoped that the present monograph will provide a useful basis for further investigation of this fascinating disorder.

2 *Clinical Aspects*

The purpose of this chapter is to provide a detailed review of those aspects of HCL that primarily concern the clinician. We have limited detailed numerical analysis of previous work to those studies giving clinical accounts of several patients [5, 16, 21, 28, 32, 40, 43, 111, 112, 149, 167, 175, 189, 202, 226, 269, 298, 322, 337, 340, 342, 373, 395]. Isolated case reports mainly concerned with a single particular aspect of the disease have been excluded and, where sequential reports have appeared from a centre, an attempt has been made to avoid including the same patient more than once. The present chapter thus reviews a total of some 500 patients, but, since the published data are often incomplete, parts of the clinical analysis are based on rather fewer patients. The personal comments included in this section are drawn from our clinical experience of 30 cases.

2.1 Occurrence

Hairy-cell leukaemia occurs in many different ethnic groups and has a wide geographic distribution, having been reported from Alaska to Japan [195, 213, 259, 370, 377]. There are no substantial epidemiological data suggesting possible aetiological factors in the disease. It has been linked with radiation exposure by reports of the disease in a nuclear-shipyard worker [273] and in a dental roentgenologist with a prolonged history of occupational radiation exposure [325]. A family with a range of malignant haematological disorders including HCL has been described, in which there was some evidence of deranged T-cell function [89], and another case with a strong family history of B-cell neoplasms has been recorded [348].

2.2 Clinical Features at Presentation

2.2.1 Age and Sex Distribution

The overall mean age at presentation is 51 years, with no marked difference between men and women (51 years for men and 48 years for women). The male : female ratio is 3.8 : 1. The detailed age and sex distribution of reported cases is given in Fig. 2.1.

2.2.2 Symptoms and Signs

Nonspecific symptoms such as weakness, weight loss, and dyspnoea are the commonest reason for presentation (75% of cases). Symptoms probably due to infection are among the presenting complaints of 28% of patients, while a haemorrhagic tendency (most often purpura, ecchymoses, or epistaxes) is complained of by 18% and abdominal symptoms referable to splenomegaly by 10%. The disease is an incidental finding in 5% of patients, while rarer reasons for presentation include rash and, very occasionally, symptomatology attributable to central nervous system involvement [298].

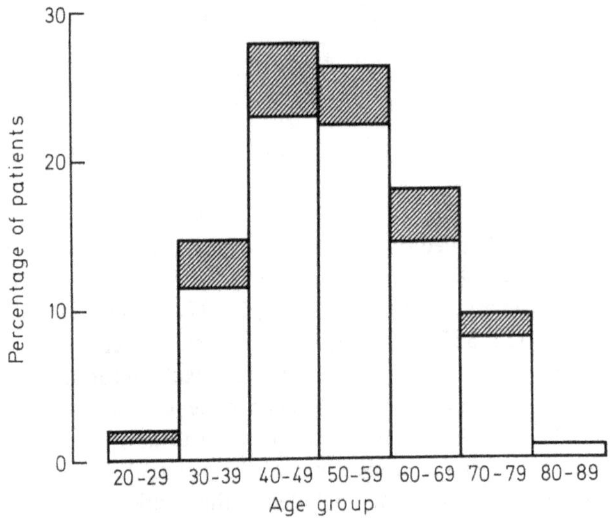

Fig. 2.1. Age and sex distribution at diagnosis. □, male; ▨, female

Splenomegaly is by far the most constant physical finding, being present in 84% of patients at presentation (> 5 cm below costal margin in 55%) and in a higher proportion at some stage of the illness [16, 269]. In our experience, discomfort caused by splenomegaly is usually relatively mild and severe pain of splenic infarction is only rarely seen.

Hepatomegaly is much less constant, being detectable in 40% of patients; hepatic enlargement is rarely marked (> 5 cm hepatomegaly is seen in only 5% of cases). In most patients there is no palpable lymphadenopathy (76%) and any lymph node enlargement is frequently limited to one node site, involving only a few small shotty glands. Even when no peripheral lymphadenopathy is present, abdominal lymphangiography will reveal abnormal para-aortic glands in a proportion of cases [16, 112, 340] (Fig. 2.2).

Maculopapular and acneiform rashes do occur but are uncommon (approximately 5%); biopsies have rarely been performed, but at least some of the maculopapular eruptions are infiltrative [149, 269]. The nature of the acneiform rash is not clear, but the lesions may be seen before the introduction of steroids [298]; this was the case in two of our patients.

2.3 Haematology at Presentation

2.3.1 Peripheral Blood

Anaemia, leucopenia and thrombocytopenia are characteristic of HCL, and pancytopenia is present in 68% of patients. The most variable parameter is the leucocyte count (Fig. 2.3).

Anaemia. Most patients are moderately anaemic and the mean Hb is similar in different large series, the overall mean being 9.8 g/dl. The range, however, is wide (2.5–17 g/dl); the distribution is shown in Fig. 2.3. The anaemia is usually described as normocytic and normochromic in type, but the mean cell volume (MCV) is nearly always towards the upper limit of normal and often definitely elevated. This macrocytosis is not accompanied by reduced serum B_{12} or folate levels or by marrow megaloblastosis. (In our series the mean

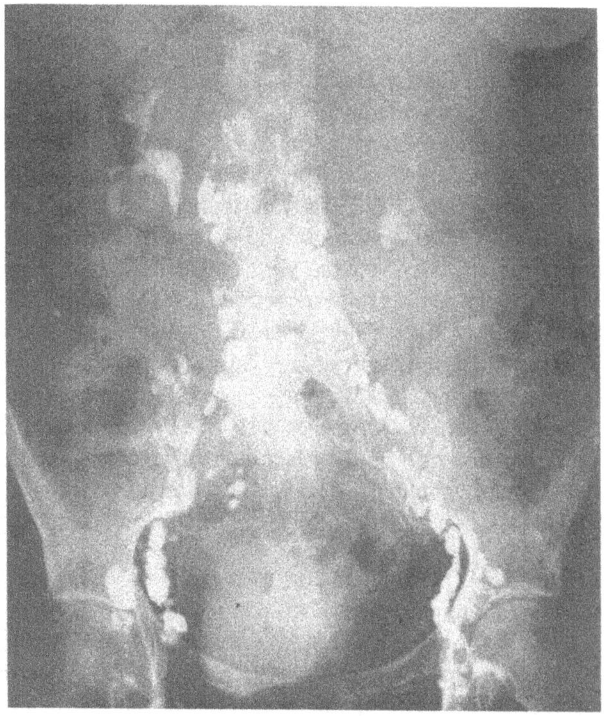

Fig. 2.2. Abdominal lymphangiogram. The lymph nodes are not markedly enlarged, but are rounder than normal and have a foamy reticulated appearance. This patient had no palpable lymphadenopathy

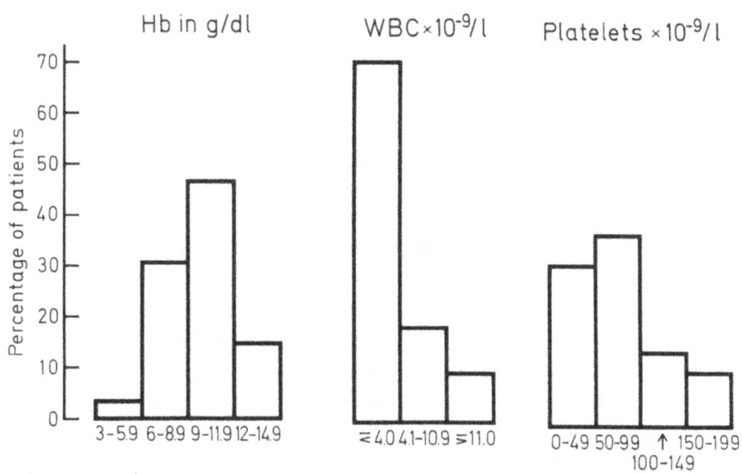

Fig. 2.3. Haematology at presentation

MCV at presentation was 100 ± 9 fl with a range of 79—123 fl, and it was > 96 fl in 70% of patients; in 90%, the MCV was repeatedly elevated at some stage of the illness.) Slight anisocytosis, poikilocytosis, and occasional circulating nucleated red cells are frequently seen, and in a few patients normoblasts may be numerous. Reticulocytosis is not a feature of the disease and haemolytic anaemia is rare. BOURONCLE et al. [29], however, have reported haemolytic anaemias with a positive antiglobulin test in six of their original patients. One of our patients developed Coombs-positive haemolytic anaemia, but this was attributed to penicillin therapy.

A number of factors contribute to the anaemia of HCL. Measurements of red-cell volume show that it is low in only about 50% of patients, the reduced Hb level in the remainder being attributable to haemodilution resulting from an increased plasma volume [62, 233]. Splenic red-cell volume and plasma volume are increased in HCL in proportion to the degree of splenomegaly [62, 233]. This increase in splenic red-cell volume is greater than that observed in other lymphoproliferative and myeloproliferative disorders with comparable splenomegaly [233], and this has been attributed to the great increase in the vascular space of the red pulp as a result of pseudosinus formation [63, 340] (Sect. 3.2).

Radiolabelling studies have revealed that in addition to splenic sequestration of red cells there is some reduction in red-cell survival in the majority of patients [40, 62, 63]. There was no correlation between this moderate haemolysis and spleen size [62].

Ferrokinetic studies have shown reduced erythropoiesis in only a minority of patients [62]. There was no evidence of ineffective erythropoiesis, and the defect appeared to be quantitative rather than qualitative. The demonstration of reduced red-cell production, even if this is only slight, is a bad prognostic feature whether or not the patient is splenectomized [62].

Leucocytes. The great majority of cases of HCL are leucopenic at presentation, but a substantial number have either a normal or an elevated leucocyte count (rarely $> 30 \times 10^9$/litre) (Fig. 2.3). The percentage of morphological HCs varies from almost nil to 100, but in general it increases with the WBC count: thus the leucopenic group (Fig. 2.3) has a mean HC score of 24%, while the groups with normal and elevated counts have 52% and 74% HCs respectively. Occasionally (7% of cases), virtually no circulating HCs are to be found in leucopenic patients.

Nearly all patients (98%) have neutropenia ($< 2.5 \times 10^9$/litre), and this is severe ($< 1 \times 10^9$/litre) in 85% and very severe ($< 0.5 \times 10^9$/litre) in 33%. Patients with elevated total WBC counts appear to be somewhat less profoundly neutropenic: there is no correlation between neutropenia and spleen size [62]. There is no corresponding deficiency of eosinophils or basophils (Sect. 6.1.2), but profound monocytopenia is nearly always present (Sect. 6.2).

Platelets. Thrombocytopenia is present in 85% of patients and is often severe (Fig. 2.3). Automated methods may sometimes yield spuriously high platelet counts, which should therefore be confirmed manually from time to time [358]. There appears to be no correlation between the leucocyte count and the severity of thrombocytopenia. Splenic sequestration is a factor in the thrombocytopenia of patients with gross splenomegaly [62, 63], but abnormal production of defective platelets is also observed [397].

2.3.2 Bone Marrow Aspiration

The bone marrow is inaspirable or yields hypocellular nondiagnostic material in 50% of cases; occasionally a dry tap at one site may be followed by successful aspiration at a second [149]. The reason for this high incidence of dry taps is not known, but it has been suggested that it may be attributable to an increase in stromal reticulin fibres or to the extensive interdigitations among infiltrating HCs [269, 373].

When marrow is successfully aspirated it is usually either normocellular or hypocellular, but it may be hypercellular. The number of infiltrating HCs varies from 5%–90%, but precise quantitation is difficult since they are frequently less "hairy" than in the peripheral blood: consequently, lymphoid cells may be conspicuous. Granulocyte and monocyte precursors are profoundly reduced, while cells of the erythroid and megakaryocytic series often appear to be relatively spared. Macrophages and plasma cells are readily found.

2.4 Other Investigations

2.4.1 Blood Chemistry

Blood urea and electrolytes and liver function tests are usually normal. In the series of GOLOMB et al. [149], raised urea (often without elevated creatinine) was observed in 30% of patients, but this has not been our experience or that of most other authors. Liver function tests are occasionally abnormal, a slightly raised alkaline phosphatase being the most usual abnormality (approximately 20% of patients). It has been suggested [70, 189] that the raised alkaline phosphatase is attributable to the periportal HC infiltration frequently present. Serum uric acid is normal.

2.4.2 Serum Proteins

In most patients serum albumin and globulin levels are normal, although decreased albumin and increased globulin are observed in some. Serum electrophoresis reveals that the raised globulin is attributable to either immunoglobulin (most commonly IgG and occasionally IgA) or $\alpha 1$ and $\alpha 2$ globulins.

Serum Immunoglobulins. Immuneparesis is rare, but hypergammaglobulinaemia is present in over 40% of cases. When immunoglobulin levels are raised there in only very rarely a monoclonal peak, although cases with paraproteinaemia have been described (Sect. 5.4.3). Autoantibody formation is not a feature of the disease.

$\beta 2$ Microglobulin. The $\beta 2$ microglobulin levels were slightly elevated in two of the seven patients tested in our series. Elevated $\beta 2$ microglobulin in the serum is a feature of both Hodgkin's and some non-Hodgkin's lymphomas [6], and probably derives from shedding by the malignant cells [6].

Serum Lysozyme. Serum lysozyme is frequently low, and is never raised.

Acute Phase Reactants. Raised $\alpha 1$ and $\alpha 2$ globulins are sometimes seen in patients who are not obviously infected, but we have found markedly elevated C-reactive protein only in a terminal patient with severe infection.

2.4.3 Erythrocyte Sedimentation Rate (ESR)

The ESR is variable in HCL, and may be either normal or elevated to high levels. Few studies have commented on the ESR in the disease, but it is our experience that marked elevation is often associated with episodes of infection.

2.4.4 Radiology

Radiological bone lesions have only rarely been observed in HCL. Skeletal surveys were performed in nine of our patients and none, including a case with paraproteinaemia, had detectable bone lesions.

A thymic mass is not found in HCL, even when the HCs possess T-cell features; mediastinal lymphadenopathy is not a feature of the disease. Abdominal lymphangiography may show para-aortic node involvement when there is no palpable lymphadenopathy; nodes may appear enlarged or simply show an abnormal distribution of dye (Fig. 2.2).

2.5 Treatment

Many patients with HCL survive in satisfactory health for prolonged periods without any therapy. Splenectomy has a definite role in the management of the disease, but other forms of treatment are of limited value.

2.5.1 Splenectomy

The precise role of splenectomy in the management of HCL is still not established and is the subject of a continuing multicentre analysis being conducted by Dr. J. Jansen in Leiden.

Splenectomy does not seem to produce improved long-term survival when all HCL patients are considered together as a group [340, 373].

Patients with absent or only minor splenomegaly have a good prognosis and do not appear to benefit from splenectomy [340]; these patients tend to be older and to have fewer circulating HCs than other patients with HCL [149]. If this group is excluded and only patients with substantial splenomegaly are considered, splenectomy is of definite statistical value, being associated with a general increase in survival and with clinical and haematological improvement in many patients [28, 63, 269, 340, 386].

In the immediate post-splenectomy period, most patients with substantial splenomegaly (90%) show an improvement in Hb and platelet levels (Fig. 2.4), and a proportion of these also show an increase in the neutrophil count. Approximately half those patients showing improvement in all three haematological parameters maintain this improvement for prolonged periods, with the Hb and platelet levels remaining within normal limits. Although the neutrophil count may improve, some asymptomatic neutropenia often persists; furthermore, the improvement in neutrophil count is frequently transient (Fig. 2.4). In the remaining patients the haematological improvement is short-lived, lasting for a period of only weeks or months.

Splenectomy need not be associated with a maintained change in the numbers of circulating HCs [149], but in a substantial number of patients a fall in peripheral blood HCs is observed [28, 340]. In approximately 10% of patients splenectomy is followed by the development of a frankly leukaemic picture (Fig. 2.4) [27, 63, 149, 340], and in some instances this may be a harbinger of clinical and haematological deterioration [63].

There is a correlation between the degree of splenic pooling and subsequent haematological improvement following splenectomy, and measurement of the splenic red-cell volume is therefore of value in the selection of patients for splenectomy [62, 233]. These are the patients in whom observed haematological abnormalities are largely attributable to splenomegaly associated with hypersplenism. In contrast, in those patients in whom the pancytopenia is very severe and associated with bone-marrow impairment, little benefit can be expected from splenectomy [63, 189]. This has been confirmed by erythrokinetic studies [62], and it seems that the demonstration of even slightly reduced erythropoiesis indicates a poor prognosis, whether or not splenectomy is performed.

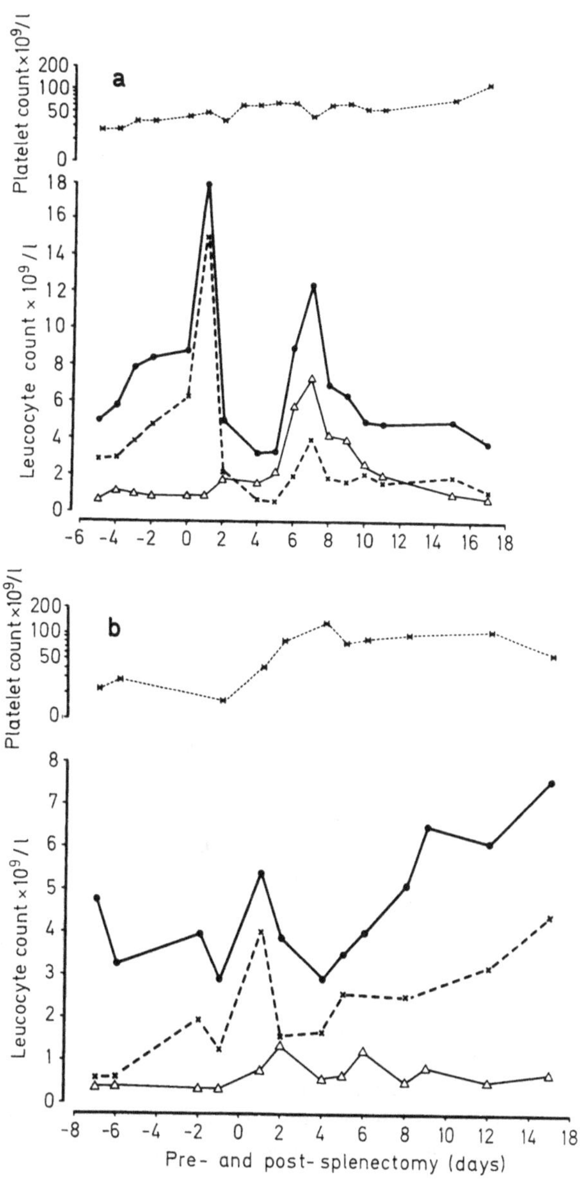

Fig. 2.4a, b. Haematology in the immediate pre- and post-splenectomy period. Both graphs illustrate the rise in total WBC count frequently observed immediately after splenectomy. This transient rise is attributable to HCs, but these cells are not simply released from the spleen during operation since the rise does not appear for several hours after this procedure [58]. |●|, platelets; ●——●, total WBC; ×- - -×, HCs; △——△, neutrophils. Patient (**a**) exemplifies the secondary rise of WBC count that may be observed on days 6–8; this rise is largely due to a transient increase in neutrophils [58]. Both patients showed a maintained improvement in platelet count, and patient (**b**) developed a floridly leukaemic picture, which was maintained for several months (but was not accompanied by clinical deterioration)

2.5.2 Chemotherapy

Steroids. The role of glucocorticoids is still disputed. Some authors have found little or no therapeutic benefit to result from their use [149, 189, 226, 298] and, particularly because of the increased risk of opportunist infection, have considered them largely contraindicated [30, 149]. It has been shown that corticosteroid alone is inferior to splenectomy in comparable groups of patients [149]. Nevertheless, steroids may sometimes be of value in the management of patients with HCL [63] by improving general well-being, reducing spleen size, and increasing the Hb level (and sometimes other haematological parameters). Thus, steroids have a place in patients too old or frail for surgery, and we have occasionally found them useful in improving the general condition of a patient immediately before splenectomy. CATOVSKY [63] has also sometimes found them to be of short-term benefit to patients in whom the response to splenectomy has been poor or who have relapsed some time after operation. There have been isolated reports of significant peripheral blood improvement following long-term administration of anabolic steroids [23, 135, 244]. However, experience with these drugs has been limited and the reported improvements were not accompanied by bone-marrow remission. Furthermore, such improvements apparently occur spontaneously in some patients, particularly after splenectomy [28, 76, 226, 348].

Cytotoxic Therapy. Most reports have agreed that cytotoxic agents, either singly or in combination, are not indicated in the chronic phase of the disease [28, 40, 202, 239, 340, 385].

Cytotoxic therapy may produce improvement, but such improvement is frequently short-lived [202, 226, 373] and therapy is accompanied by the risk of exacerbating existing cytopenia and of further compromising the immune system [385]. Even so, a trial of nonaggressive chemotherapy is probably indicated in patients slowly deteriorating after splenectomy followed by steroids. What chemotherapeutic agent should be used in this context is not clear: vincristine and alkylating agents may sometimes be of value [63, 146a], but 6-mercaptopurine has not been found beneficial [145].

Induction of complete remission by aggressive cytotoxic chemotherapy has been described [100, 250, 393], but combination therapy may fail and remissions have only occurred after prolonged marrow depression during which the patients required vigorous supportive measures. Therefore, aggressive chemotherapy is only warranted in deteriorating patients who have severely compromised bone-marrow function and have already failed to respond to splenectomy followed by nonaggressive chemotherapy. At exactly what stage the risk of aggressive cytotoxics becomes justified is a fine point of judgment; but severe, progressive, and symptomatic neutropenia carries a bad prognosis [340] and its presence should perhaps encourage an aggressive policy. There are insufficient data to suggest the optimal therapeutic regimen, although cytosine arabinoside and the anthracyclines appear to be active agents [100, 250].

Lithium. Lithium produces an increase in the peripheral neutrophil count both in normal subjects and in patients rendered neutropenic by cytotoxic therapy [81, 362]. This appears to be an indirect effect resulting from the ability of lithium to enhance colony-stimulating activity [168]. We have tested the effect of lithium carbonate (1,000–2,000 mg/day to produce a serum level approximately equal to 1 mEq/litre for at least 28 days) on the neutropenia of HCL in three patients. No consistent elevation of neutrophil count was observed.

2.5.3 Irradiation

Despite the fact that HCs are resistant to radiation in vitro [339], splenic irradiation can sometimes be of value in ameliorating the symptoms of the disease, in reducing spleen size, and, occasionally, in improving haematological parameters [28, 373]. However, no benefit may ensue [28, 202], and any improvement achieved is usually short-lived [202, 373]. The treatment is sometimes associated with severe marrow depression [28, 202, 373]; the mechanism of this myelosuppression is not clear, but it is possible to postulate release of a myelotoxic factor from the irradiated spleen.

Radiation to specific areas of HC infiltration may be indicated if these are causing symptoms. For example, irradiation has proved effective, when chemotherapy had failed, in abolishing

chylous ascitic and pleural effusions complicating the disease [97]. Similarly, irradiation has produced relief of bone pain associated with lytic lesions [373].
^{32}P therapy has been tried, but appears to yield no benefit [28, 298].

2.6 Clinical and Haematological Progress

2.6.1 Survival and Prognostic Features

HCL is usually a chronic disorder, but may run an acute or subacute course. The median survival in the disease is of the order of 50 months. The range is very wide and patients have survived for as long as 27 years. Approximately 40% of patients die within 2 years of diagnosis, irrespective of treatment. After 2 years the death rate is much reduced, and the overall 5- and 10-year survival rates are of the order of 50% and 35% respectively.
The effect of splenomegaly and of therapy on prognosis has been considered in the previous section (Sect. 2.5). Other factors influencing prognosis have been considered by SEBAHOUN et al. [340]. Sex (men fare slightly worse than women) and the presence of a leucocytosis possibly indicate a poorer prognosis, whereas thrombocytopenia ($< 50 \times 10^9$/litre), mild anaemia (< 12 g/dl), lymphocyte count, serum γ-globulin level, and marrow cellularity are all devoid of any statistically significant prognostic value. Progressive marrow impairment, reflected in profound neutropenia and severe anaemia, is a major prognostic feature; the demonstration of even slightly reduced erythropoiesis is of serious prognostic significance, the majority of patients displaying this feature being dead in less than a year [62].

2.6.2 Course and Fluctuations in the Disease

The course of the illness is variable. Many patients remain relatively well for prolonged periods. Other patients, having been stable for a variable time, steadily decline and die after suffering repeated infections and after requiring multiple blood transfusions. In another group of patients the course is acute or subacute from the outset [189, 373]. Still others display a fluctuating course with periods of exacerbation (recurrent infections and progressive anaemia), followed by periods of marked improvement. Such fluctuations may be related to therapy or to infection (see Sect. 2.7.1), but remissions sometimes appear to occur spontaneously [28, 226, 348].
We have attempted to analyse these fluctuations by performing a sequential immunological surface-marker study of the peripheral blood cells of a group of ten patients, and by correlating the results with the clinical and haematological progress of the patients [76]. In four cases no major change in peripheral populations was observed, and HCs with a B-cell phenotype remained prominent throughout the period of study (Fig. 2.5a). These patients had consistent anaemia, neutropenia, monocytopenia, and thrombocytopenia, but remained relatively stable without recurrent infection or the need for transfusion. Two of them had undergone splenectomy, two had not. One had received continuous steroid medication throughout the period of follow-up, and one had a severe chest infection requiring hospitalization.
In the remaining six patients there was a complete reversal in the major peripheral blood cell type from morphological HCs with a B-cell phenotype to lymphoid cells with a T-cell phenotype. This reversal (Fig. 2.5b–d), which was transient in two of the patients (Fig. 2.5b, c), was accompanied by marked symptomatic and haematological improvement in five, and improvement was not observed without this reversal in predominant cell population.

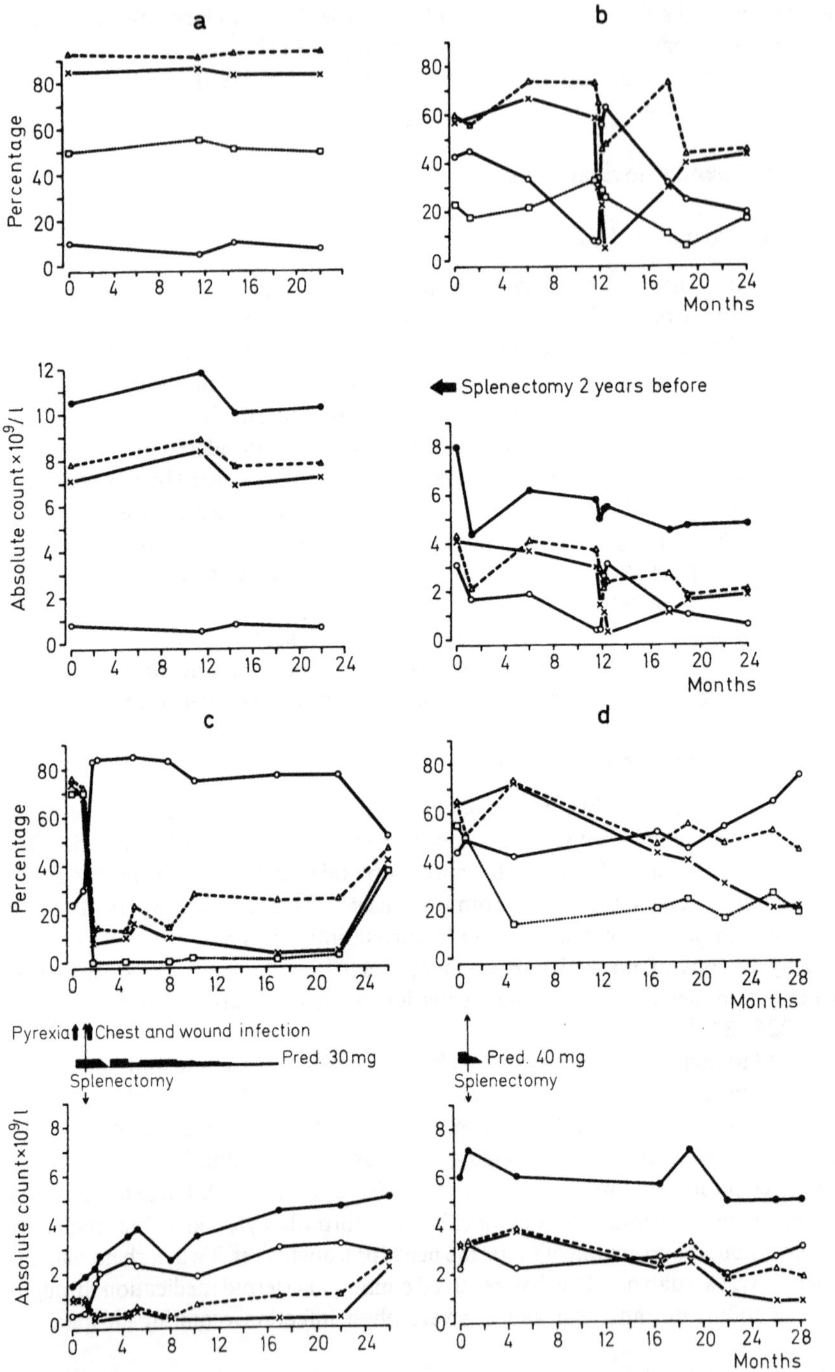
a
b
Percentage
Months
Absolute count ×10⁹/l
Splenectomy 2 years before
c
d
Pyrexia
Chest and wound infection
Pred. 30 mg
Splenectomy
Pred. 40 mg
Splenectomy

Fig. 2.5a–d

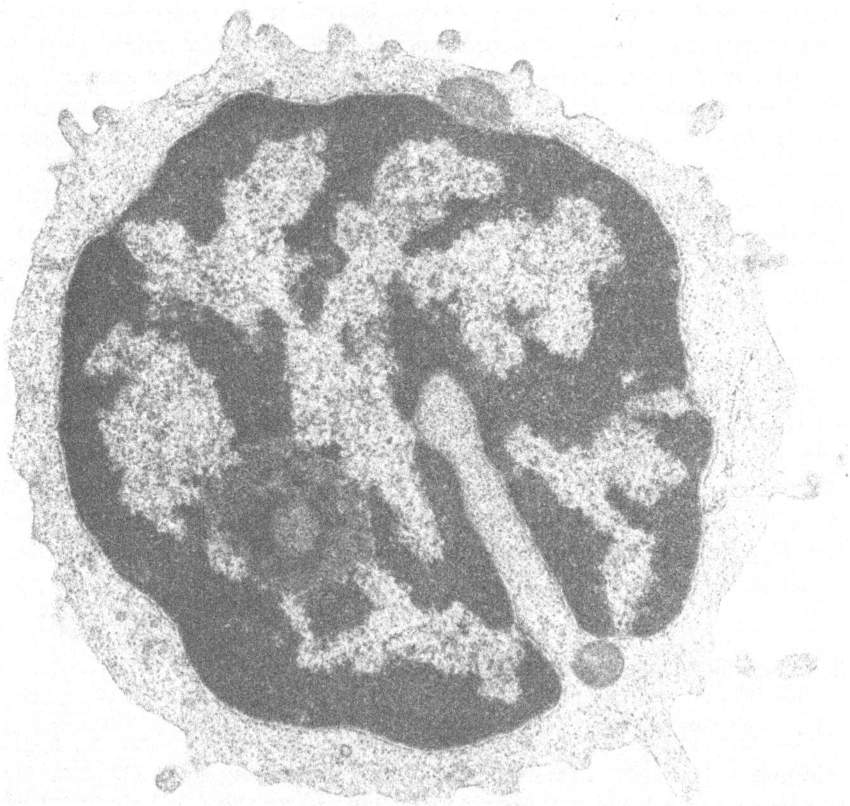

Fig. 2.6. Notched cells in the T-cell phase of HCL. The striking indentation of the nucleus is illustrated. The nucleus appears mature in containing heavily condensed peripheral chromatin, and is typical in possessing a well-developed nucleolus. The high nuclear: cytoplasmic ratio of the cells is clearly shown (× 21,000)

◂ **Fig. 2.5a–d.** Fluctuations in the peripheral blood during the course of HCL in four patients. ●—●, total WBC count; □···□, % HCs; △---△, γFc receptor-bearing cells; ○—○, E-rosetting cells; ×——×, SIg-bearing cells. Rosetting cells are graphed as percentages of mononuclear cells (*upper graph* for each patient) and in absolute values (*lower graph* for each patient). **a** Illustrates an example of a patient who remained stable for a prolonged period, the peripheral cell populations remaining substantially unchanged. **b** Shows a patient in whom there was a transient reversal in the predominant cell population, with E-rosetting T cells forming the major peripheral blood cell population for a short period. This transient change was associated with prolonged clinical improvement. **c** Represents a patient in whom the reversal of cell populations occurred immediately after splenectomy; HCs virtually disappeared and there was an absolute increase in the numbers of circulating T cells. The change was maintained for a prolonged period and throughout this period the patient remained in excellent health. Clinical relapse coincided with the reappearance of HCs as the predominant cell type. **d** Shows a patient in whom, although HCs became reduced immediately after splenectomy, the reversal of major cell populations (with T cells becoming predominant) occurred apparently spontaneously some 2 years after splenectomy. This T-cell phase with HCs present in only small numbers was again associated with excellent health

The therapeutic circumstances of the reversal differed, but splenectomy probably played some part, since clinical and haematological improvement immediately followed the procedure in two patients and was not observed in patients who had not undergone splenectomy. The reversal could not be directly related to chemotherapy or infection, and in two patients it appeared to occur spontaneously 2–3 years after splenectomy. The persistent neutropenia and the continued presence of disease in the bone marrow, together with the demonstration of several morphological and immunological abnormalities in the circulating T cells, suggested that these changes did not constitute complete remission. For example, in most patients the "T-cell phase" was associated with a modest elevation above normal of the absolute T-cell count. The T cells were strikingly notched (Fig. 2.6), most failed to express receptors for the Fc of IgM or IgG after culture (see Sect. 6.4.1), and reduced numbers displayed the dot esterase staining pattern characteristically present in the majority of normal T lymphocytes [161, 176]. In addition, the T cells, unlike normal T lymphocytes [24] but like some lymphomatous T cells [230], showed a lack of concordance in their dot-staining pattern with esterase and acid phosphatase. Finally, and perhaps most importantly, the T cells in three of four cases tested during this T-cell phase contained intracytoplasmic IgD. All these points suggested that the T-cell phase did not simply represent the re-emergence of the normal T-cell component of peripheral blood, but rather that the lymphoid cells are directly involved in the clonal proliferation [76].

2.7 Complications and Cause of Death

2.7.1 Infections

Infection is the major cause of morbidity and mortality in HCL. Of more than 200 documented deaths covered in our review, infection was recorded as the terminal event in 63%. Bronchopneumonia and septicaemia are by far the most common fatal infections, together accounting for 84% of infectious deaths. The causative organism, where isolated, is usually a gram-negative bacillus, with *Ps. aeruginosa* accounting for an unusually high proportion of infections. Bacterial sepsis is sometimes accompanied by disseminated fungal infection (2%) or by viraemia (1%). The remaining infectious deaths have been attributed to disseminated or pulmonary fungal/yeast infections (7%) caused by *Aspergillus fumigatus* or *Candida albicans* or to meningitis caused by *Cryptococcus neoformans*. Tuberculosis is recorded as the cause of death in 7% of cases and occasionally atypical mycobacteria have been implicated. Terminal viral hepatitis, probably associated with transfusion, has been described in 2% of cases.

Bouza et al. [30] have recently reviewed the incidence and cause of infections in HCL. At presentation, 28% of patients have some infection and this rises to over 60% during the course of the disease. Bacterial pneumonia and septicaemia account for the majority of infectious episodes, and *Ps. aeruginosa* and *E. coli* are most frequently the causative organisms. There is clear evidence [30, 149] that the incidence of infectious episodes correlates with the absolute neutrophil count and that counts of less than 0.5×10^9/litre strongly predispose to infection. Patients who have undergone splenectomy have fewer infections [30], and this is probably at least partly attributable to the quantitative and qualitative improvements in neutrophils that may follow this procedure (Sect. 6.1.1). (Immediate post-operative infections are frequently observed.) Although corticosteroid administration is associated with an increased risk of potentially life-threatening fungal infection [30], its statistical correlation with other infections is not convincing [149].

Opportunistic infections are frequent and have been observed before the instigation of any chemotherapy. The list of the ubiquitous organisms that have been isolated from HCL provides an almost comprehensive catalogue of opportunistic agents. The following have all been recorded: *Herpes simplex* [63, 202]; cytomegalovirus [43]; disseminated *Aspergillus fumigatus* [202]; *Candida albicans* [340]; *Histoplasma capsulatum* [28, 149]; meningeal *Cryptococcus neoformans* [28, 342]; *Pneumocystis carinii* [28]; *Toxoplasma gondii* [112]. Tuberculosis is an important and frequent infection in HCL, and the infection can rarely be attributed to prior chemotherapy. Typical pulmonary tuberculosis is not unusual [28, 63, 248], but the incidence of atypical mycobacterial infection is higher than in malignancies in general [378]. Several cases in which slowly growing atypical mycobacteria have been isolated have now been described [28, 60, 173, 247, 378]. Mycobacteria from Runyon's groups I, II, and III have all been found, but *M. kansasii* (Runyon's group I) has been isolated most frequently. Atypical mycobacterial infection may present a considerable diagnostic problem [60]. Skin testing with PPD is usually negative, although HCL patients are capable of yielding a positive response to PPD [60], and mycobacteria are rarely isolated from sputum, urine, blood, or bone marrow until late in the disease. Several authors have commented on the importance of liver or lymph-node biopsy for diagnosis [60, 248, 378]; for although the disease is frequently disseminated, it is occasionally localized to the lungs and lymph nodes [173]. This difficulty in diagnosis means that the incidence of atypical mycobacterial infection may be even higher than has been recorded, and the unresponsive fever of unknown origin (PUO) frequently described in HCL [30, 63, 337] may sometimes be undiagnosed mycobacterial infection. For example, Marie et al. [248] recorded that four of their patients with PUO became afebrile on antituberculous therapy, and one of our patients with PUO, who was treated empirically with antituberculous drugs, also responded. Our patient had a delayed response to treatment, and this has also been the experience of others employing a combination antituberculous drug regimen [378]. Failure of PUO to respond to antituberculous therapy does not rule out atypical mycobacterial infection, since most proven cases of atypical tuberculosis have not responded and have died of the disease, and in vitro testing may show extreme resistance to most drugs [173, 378]. Therefore, in cases of HCL with PUO, liver biopsy (or node biopsy) should be considered and material sent for culture as well as for histology.

It has been suggested that the monocytopenia and defective monocyte function of HCL (Sect. 6.2) are important in predisposing to disseminated mycobacterial infection [28, 378]. However, defective T-cell function, together with the possibility that weakly phagocytic but nonmicrobicidal HCs disseminate the organism without priming T cells, are also factors that may be important and are perhaps worth further investigation.

Infection and/or trauma may be capable of inducing important cellular changes in the disease. For example, we have observed a patient who was floridly leukaemic after splenectomy, but then suffered a pyrexial illness during which the circulating HCs disappeared and the total WBC count returned to normal. The majority of circulating mononuclear cells during this period possessed receptors for the Fc of IgG, but lacked SIg and did not form E rosettes. After the pyrexial episode, typical HCs with the normal marker phenotype (Sect. 5.5) reappeared. We have also observed a patient in whom HCs disappeared from the peripheral blood shortly after a major head injury.

2.7.2 Noninfectious Complications

After infection, bleeding is the most serious complication of HCL. Haemorrhage is frequently associated with infection, but is only occasionally (8%) the major cause of death. During the course of the illness, the most common haemorrhagic manifestations are skin purpura or ecchymoses, although epistaxes and bleeding from other sites can occur.

A variety of other complications can occasionally arise. Splenic rupture has been recorded but is rare [28, 167, 320, 340, 373]. Involvement of nonlymphoreticular sites very occasionally gives rise to skin [62, 149] and meningeal disease [298]. Chylous and serous ascitic and pleural effusions have been recorded [97, 219], and HCs may be identifiable in these [219]. Localized bone disease causing lytic bone lesions associated with pain has been documented [313, 373].

An unusual association, which may be due to more than chance, is the occurrence of polyarteritis nodosa in HCL [183], and we ourselves have had one patient with veno-occlusive disease of the lung and associated fibrosing alveolitis in which immune complex deposition may have played a part.

Several instances of second tumour in HCL have been recorded [28, 40, 43, 149, 298, 337]; these have involved a variety of histological tumour types at different sites. It is not known whether HCL, like chronic lymphocytic leukaemia (CLL) [145], is associated with an increased risk of second tumour formation.

3 Pathology

A wide range of sites and tissues may be involved clinically (Sect. 2.7) or at post-mortem [28, 373], but the major sites of infiltration are organs of the lymphoreticular system, including the bone marrow.

3.1 Bone Marrow

The bone marrow is always involved in HCL, and its histology is diagnostic [39, 376]. Although it is our experience that at least a few HCs are always to be found in the peripheral blood at presentation, bone biopsy material can sometimes be the means by which a diagnosis is initially made [39]. In this regard, both the histology of the marrow [39] and the tartrate-resistant acid phosphatase (TRAP) staining of imprint preparations of the bone biopsy may be of value [221].

Burke [39] has described the diagnostic histological appearances in some detail. The mononuclear-cell infiltration may be partial or complete (in almost equal numbers of cases), but is always diffuse. The apparently focal infiltration described in HCL [373] is attributable to the fact that, in partial marrow involvement, the HC infiltration of residual haematopoietic islands may be inconspicuous [39] and the marrow normocellular. In complete involvement the marrow is hypercellular, fat spaces are largely obliterated, and the infiltrate is seen as a monotonous sheet of relatively widely spaced mononuclear cells [39, 269, 373]. Few mitoses are seen. In both partial and complete infiltrations the mononuclear cells, although they do not display obvious cytoplasmic hairs, nevertheless present a distinctive appearance in which the well-defined nuclei are separated from one another by a clear zone of cytoplasm or occasionally by clear spaces, imparting what has been described as a halo appearance (Fig. 3.1). This appearance has been attributed to the relatively abundant cytoplasm possessed by HCs, but also to shrinkage artifact [39, 373]. When involvement is complete, virtually no residual myelopoiesis is observed. When involvement is partial, the residual haematopoietic islands are composed predominantly of cells of the erythroid and megakaryocytic series. Granulopoiesis is usually profoundly depressed, but a case with both granulocytic and megakaryocytic hyperplasia has been described [39]. Mature plasma cells and macrophages are not uncommon (Fig. 3.2), and we have observed two patients in whom macrophages were very prominent.

In most patients, no major quantitative or qualitative changes are observed over a prolonged period, but both progression [167] and, less commonly, regression of the cellularity can occur, and such changes may be related to splenectomy [39].

There is general agreement [40, 70, 111, 221, 269, 337, 373] that reticulin fibres are increased, whether marrow involvement is partial or complete [39]. The cause of this reticulin fibrosis is unknown, but fibroblasts can be identified interspersed among the HCs [376]. Occasionally, "fibroblastic change" (focal collections of uniform fusiform cells with vesicular nuclei) has been recorded [8, 39, 269, 373], and this change has been related to the increase in reticulin fibres.

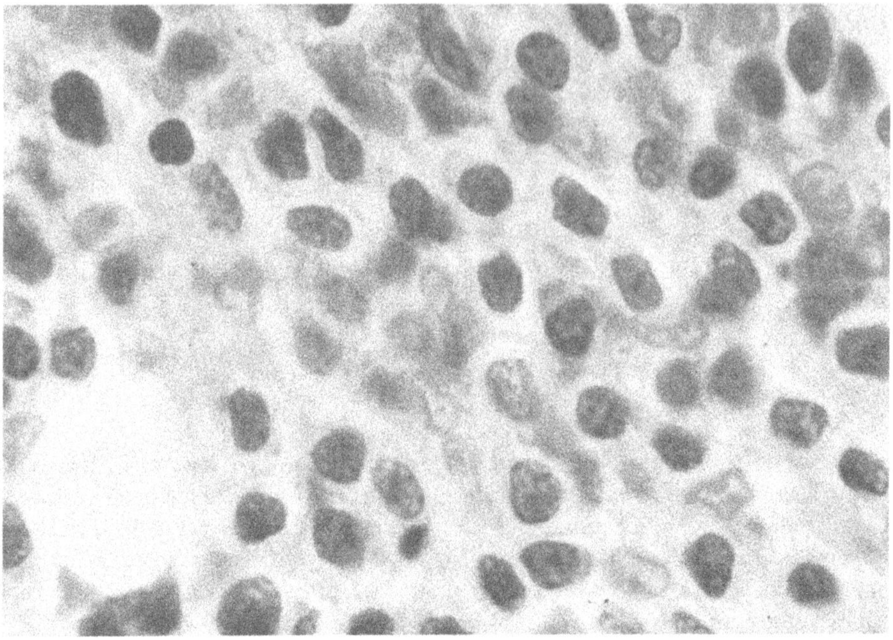

Fig. 3.1. Bone biopsy. H and E stain. The marrow is diffusely infiltrated by widely spaced HCs, imparting a halo appearance

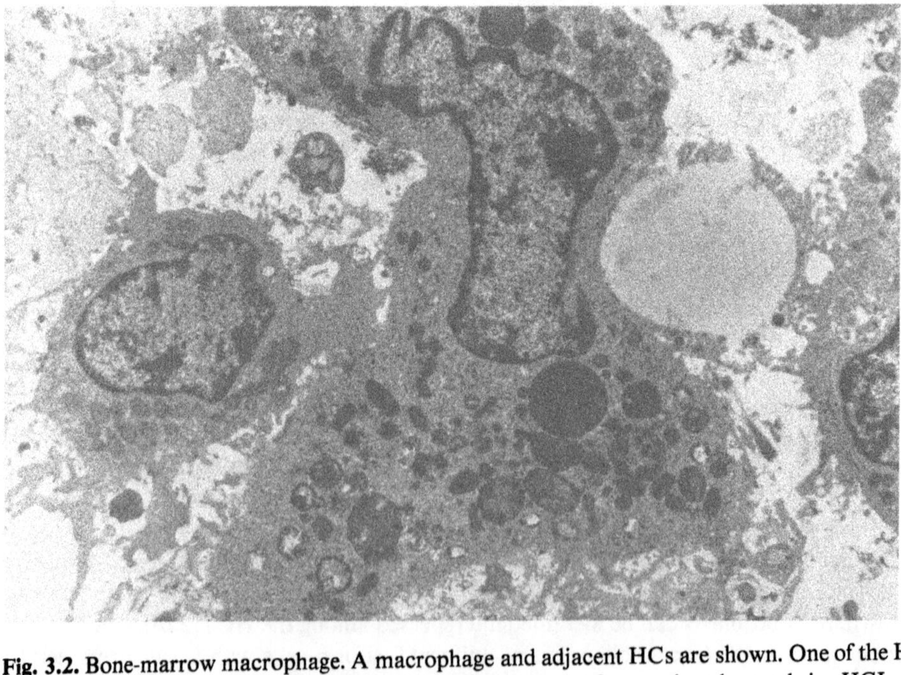

Fig. 3.2. Bone-marrow macrophage. A macrophage and adjacent HCs are shown. One of the HCs is closely interdigitating with the macrophage and this is frequently observed in HCL [139] (× 6,000)

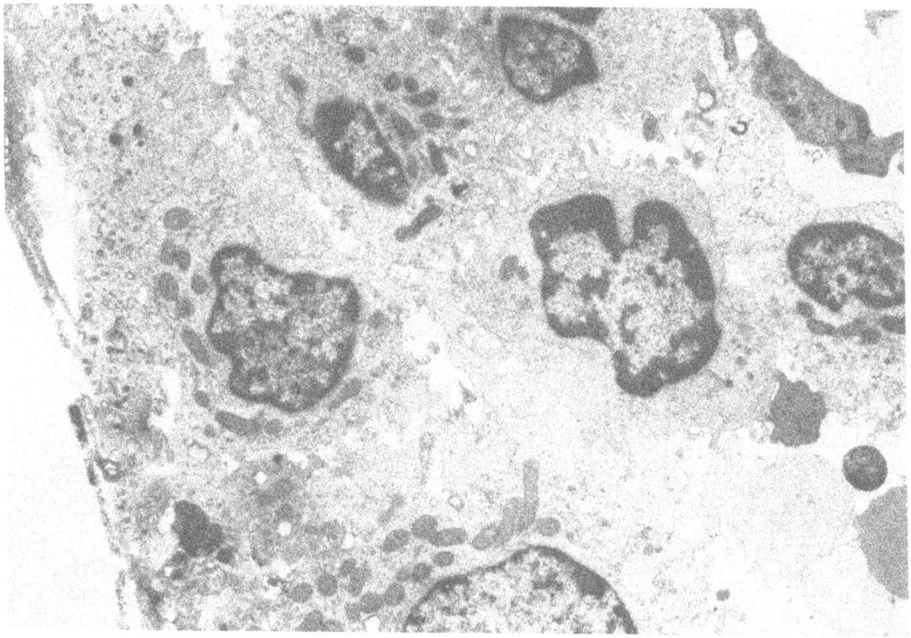

Fig. 3.3. Bone marrow. The marrow is replaced by loosely interdigitating HCs. Fat spaces are seen at either side of the micrograph (× 5,000)

Mature collagen is frequently absent or minimal [269, 373], but has been reported to be increased in some cases [111, 203].
Electron microscopy confirms the HC nature of the infiltrate [203]. Extensive interdigitations between adjoining HCs are apparent, but the cells are frequently less closely packed than in spleen fixed in an identical manner and spaces are often present between adjoining cells (Fig. 3.3). In other ways the cells do not differ from those in the peripheral blood; in particular, when ribosome-lamella (R-L) complexes are present in peripheral blood HCs they are also to be found in the infiltrating marrow cells.

3.2 Spleen

The spleen is variably enlarged and generally weights between 350 and 5,000 g [40, 70, 109, 202, 269]. The tissue is of a firm consistency (Fig. 3.4), and its cut surface presents a homogeneous dark-red appearance with no evidence of circumscribed tumour; Malpighian bodies are atrophic or absent (Fig. 3.4). Areas of recent or healed infarction have been reported, but their frequency has varied in different reports [28, 40, 202, 373].
Imprint preparations reveal large numbers of mononuclear cells with a nucleus and cytoplasm resembling those of peripheral blood HCs. The mononuclear cells contain strong TRAP activity but lack the characteristic surface projections of peripheral HCs.
Histological examination shows diffuse infiltration of the red pulp by mononuclear cells containing slightly irregular nuclei with fine stippled chromatin; nucleoli are not prominent and mitoses are not seen (Fig. 3.5). The white pulp is either totally obliterated or seen as small

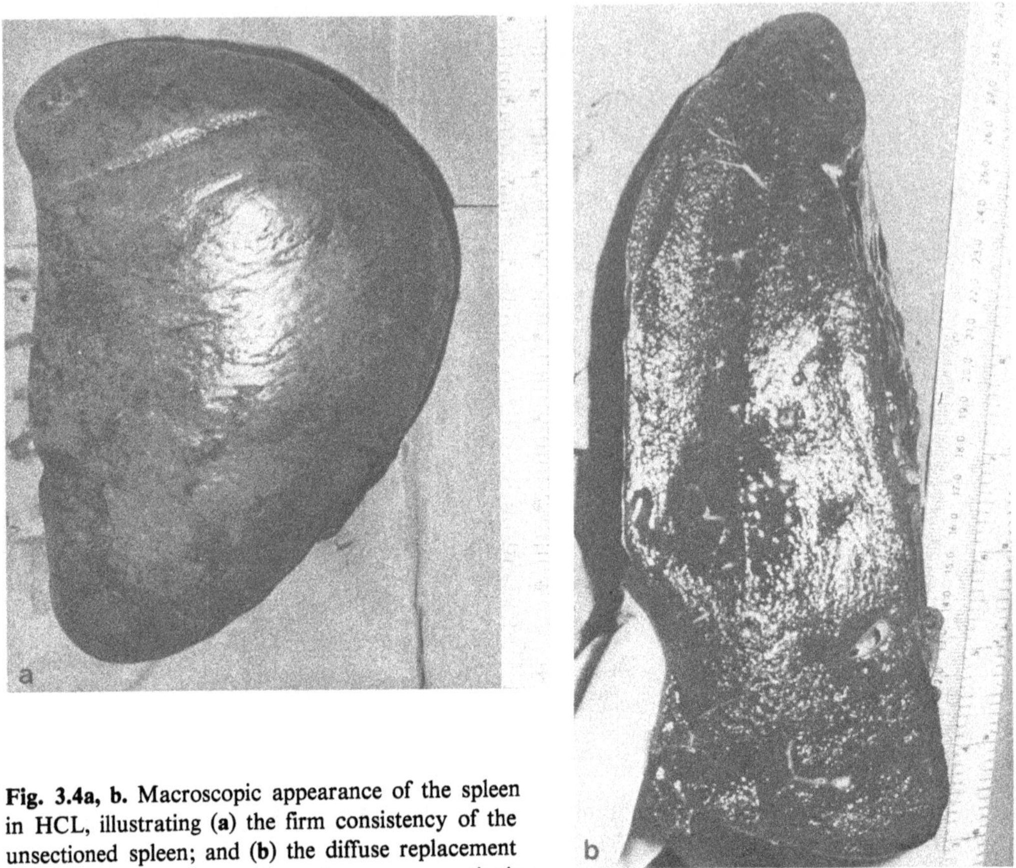

Fig. 3.4a, b. Macroscopic appearance of the spleen in HCL, illustrating (**a**) the firm consistency of the unsectioned spleen; and (**b**) the diffuse replacement and obliteration of the white pulp seen on sectioning

atrophic lymphoid follicles without germinal centres, while periarterial lymphoid sheaths are absent [40, 276]. The capsule and trabeculae are not infiltrated.

The red pulp is so heavily infiltrated with HCs that it is frequently difficult to distinguish cords and sinuses. In certain areas variably sized blood-filled spaces lined by HCs, rather than endothelial cells, are to be seen in at least the great majority of cases [114, 115, 269, 275, 276, 373] (Fig. 3.5). These structures, which have been termed pseudoangiomatous dilatations of sinuses [114, 115] or pseudosinuses [275, 276], may appear singly or in clusters [275, 276] presenting a haemangiomatous appearance [275]. NANBA et al. [275, 276] established the HC nature of the cells lining the pseudosinuses by demonstrating that these cells contained TRAP but lacked naphthyl AS-D acetate esterase (a marker of endothelial cells). The ring fibres that surround normal splenic sinuses are absent from pseudosinuses, but the reticulin fibres of the splenic cords persist (Fig. 3.5) and are frequently increased. Pseudosinus formation appears to be a progressive infiltrative process, since partial pseudosinus formation may be observed in which residual endothelial cells can be identified morphologically and histochemically; such sinuses may be surrounded by attenuated ring fibres.

In addition to large numbers of HCs, the splenic cords contain readily identifiable macrophages, plasma cells, and spindle-shaped cells with a compact nucleus. The macrophages contain phagocytosed cell debris and are particularly well visualized by nonspecific esterase

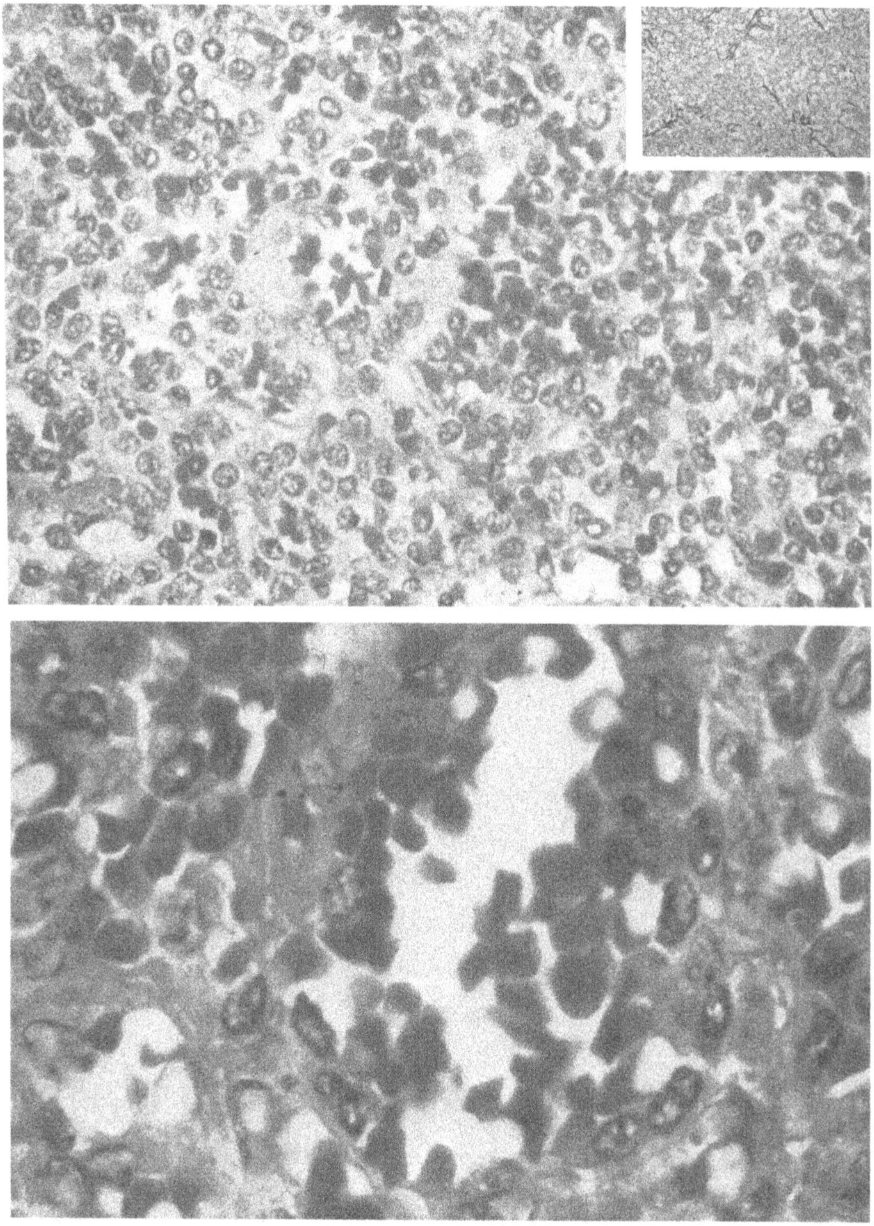

Fig. 3.5. Histology of the spleen. H and E preparation; *inset* reticulin stain. Vascular spaces lined mainly by HCs are evident. The *inset* shows that reticulin is prominent in the splenic cords, but is sparse around the sinuses

(NSE) staining or by immunoperoxidase methods detecting phagocytosed immunoglobulin [153] (Fig. 3.6). We also employed this last method to demonstrate that the plasma cells from 11 spleens did not show monoclonal light chain involvement and were therefore presumably reactive [153]. In addition to being scattered throughout the splenic cords, plasma cells often appear to be particularly numerous around blood vessels [153] (Fig. 3.6). The spindle-shaped

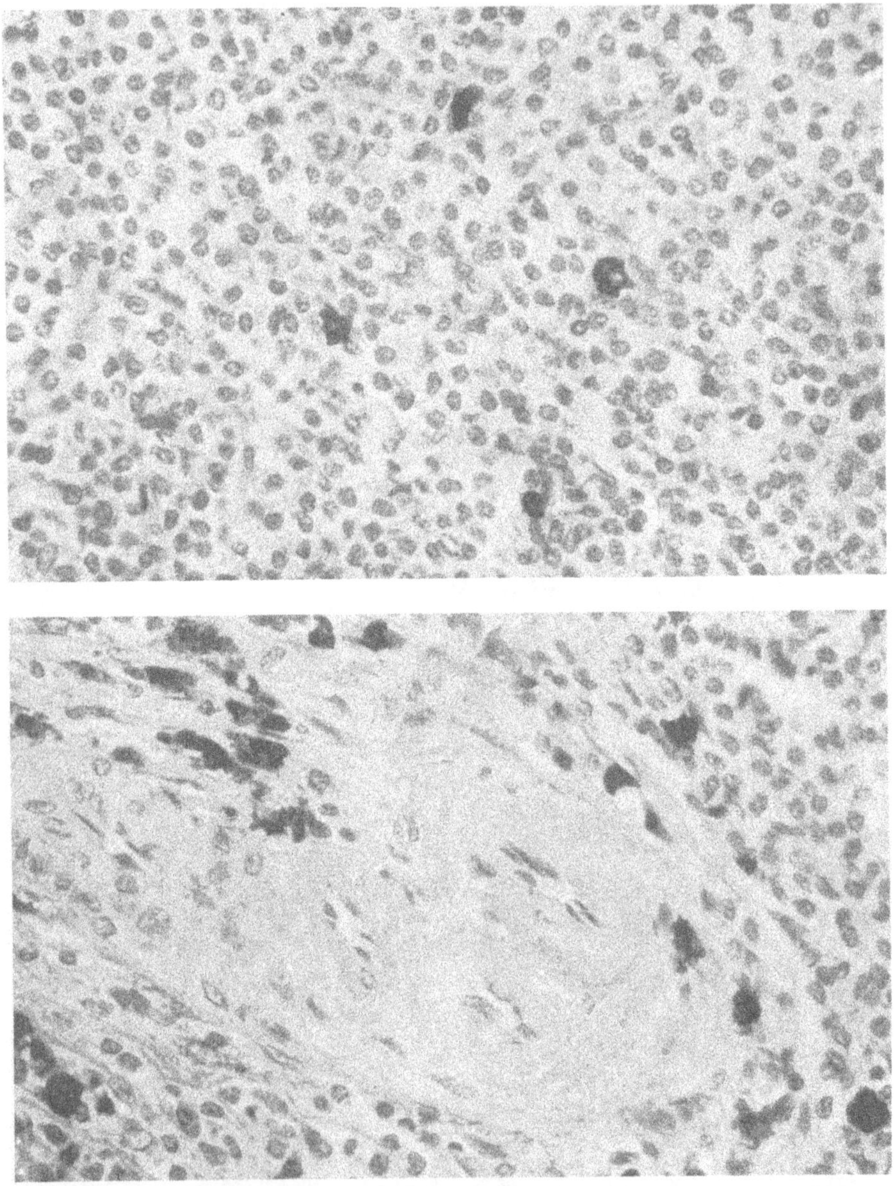

Fig. 3.6. Histology of the spleen. Immunoperoxidase stain. In the *upper panel*, four strongly reactive plasma cells are seen. The numerous infiltrating HCs are unreactive; HCs can be shown to contain Ig by other techniques, and this lack of reactivity is probably attributable to damage during fixation and processing [153]. In the *lower panel*, the Ig-positive cells surrounding the blood vessels are numerous and consist of both plasma cells and macrophages

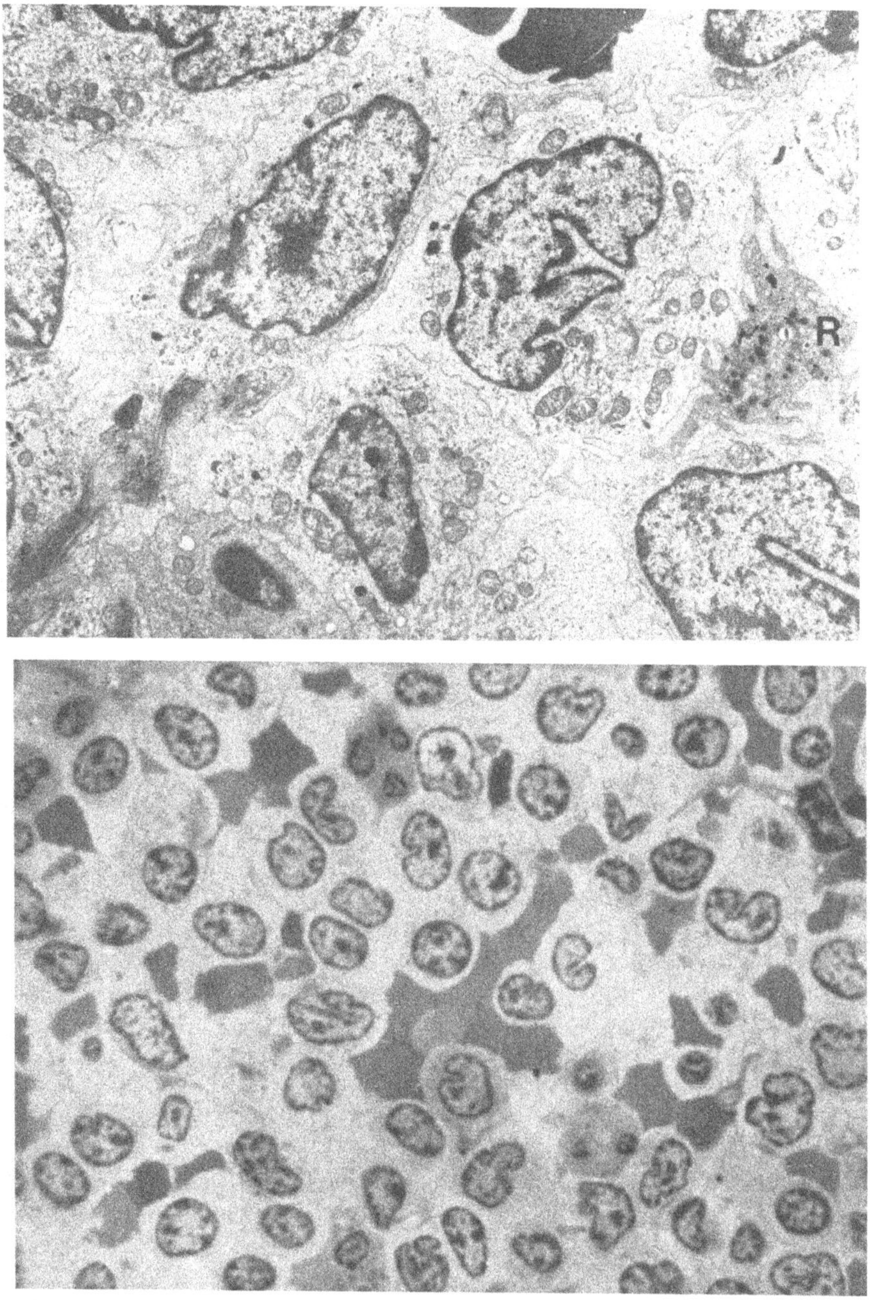

Fig. 3.7. Splenic ultrastructure. Many closely interdigitating HCs are seen. One reticuloendothelial cell (*R*) is present. The semithin section stained with toluidine blue shows the diffuse infiltration by HCs which surround the small vascular spaces. Some positively stained R-L complexes can be visualized in this preparation (× 5,500)

cells have been shown to be intimately associated with reticulin fibres [276], and are possibly the cells responsible for their production. Extramedullary haematopoiesis is infrequent, but is occasionally observed [276].

Ultrastructural study [28, 41] has added little to basic histological observations, but has shown that surface projections are readily evident on the infiltrating mononuclear cells (Fig. 3.7), despite their apparent absence in histological and imprint preparations. The precise appearance of these surface projections depends upon the degree of packing of the HCs. When packing is loose the hairs are relatively more prominent, but when the HCs are tightly packed the surface projections are seen as complex interdigitations (Fig. 3.7) and the infiltrating cells present a syncytium-like appearance [41]. BURKE et al. [41] have also observed cytoplasmic projections of HCs protruding between sinusoidal endothelial cells and fenestrations of the underlying basal lamina.

The histological appearance of the spleen with primary involvement of the red pulp is of a type seen in monocytic proliferations [40], and is quite different from that observed in most B-cell lymphomas. This picture is largely diagnostic [40], and the identification of pseudosinus formation is a further diagnostic point in HCL [275]. The pseudosinus formation is probably responsible for the prominent splenic red-cell pooling of the disease (Sect. 2.3.1). The frequency of splenic macrophages is of interest in view of the peripheral monocytopenia in HCL [53, 274], but the influence of these macrophages on the pancytopenia of the disease seems to be relatively minor.

3.3 Liver

Exceptions have been reported [28], but the liver is nearly always variably infiltrated by HCs and its weight is frequently increased to 2,500 g or more [40, 70, 202, 269, 373]. At the time of splenectomy, the liver surface appears grossly normal, but at autopsy small nodular areas of infiltration may be seen in cut sections [202].

Histological examination shows a mononuclear cell infiltration of both the sinusoids and the portal tracts, but the general architecture of the liver remains intact (Fig. 3.8). In a minority of cases the infiltration is relatively slight, involving only the sinusoids, and may be misinterpreted as Kupffer-cell hyperplasia [104]. More frequently, sinusoidal involvement is prominent and the HCs may lie free within the lumen or in close association with the endothelium and adjacent hepatocytes [104]. Ultrastructural studies have shown that the HCs actually attach to the sinusoidal wall by means of cytoplasmic processes in a manner closely resembling Kupffer-cell attachment [104, 107].

Portal tract involvement may take the form of angiomatous lesions composed of dilated spaces lined by HCs and filled with erythrocytes [114, 115, 275]. Although they resemble pseudosinuses, these lesions are less constant than in the spleen [104, 275, 373]. The angiomatous lesions are encircled by thick reticulin fibres, which are continuous with those of the hepatic sinusoids [275]. The lesions are usually confined to the portal tracts [114, 115, 275] and only occasionally extend into the adjacent hepatic parenchyma [275]. However, small similar isolated lesions with associated reticulin fibres may occasionally be observed within the hepatic sinusoids. Plasma cells are not infrequent, particularly in the portal tracts, and (as in the spleen) these are reactive [153].

In view of this extensive involvement of the liver, the relatively minor clinical enlargement of this organ in the disease is perhaps surprising. Nor is it clear why hepatocyte structure and function are so well preserved. Nevertheless, hepatic histology, like that of the spleen and bone marrow, is diagnostic of the disease [104].

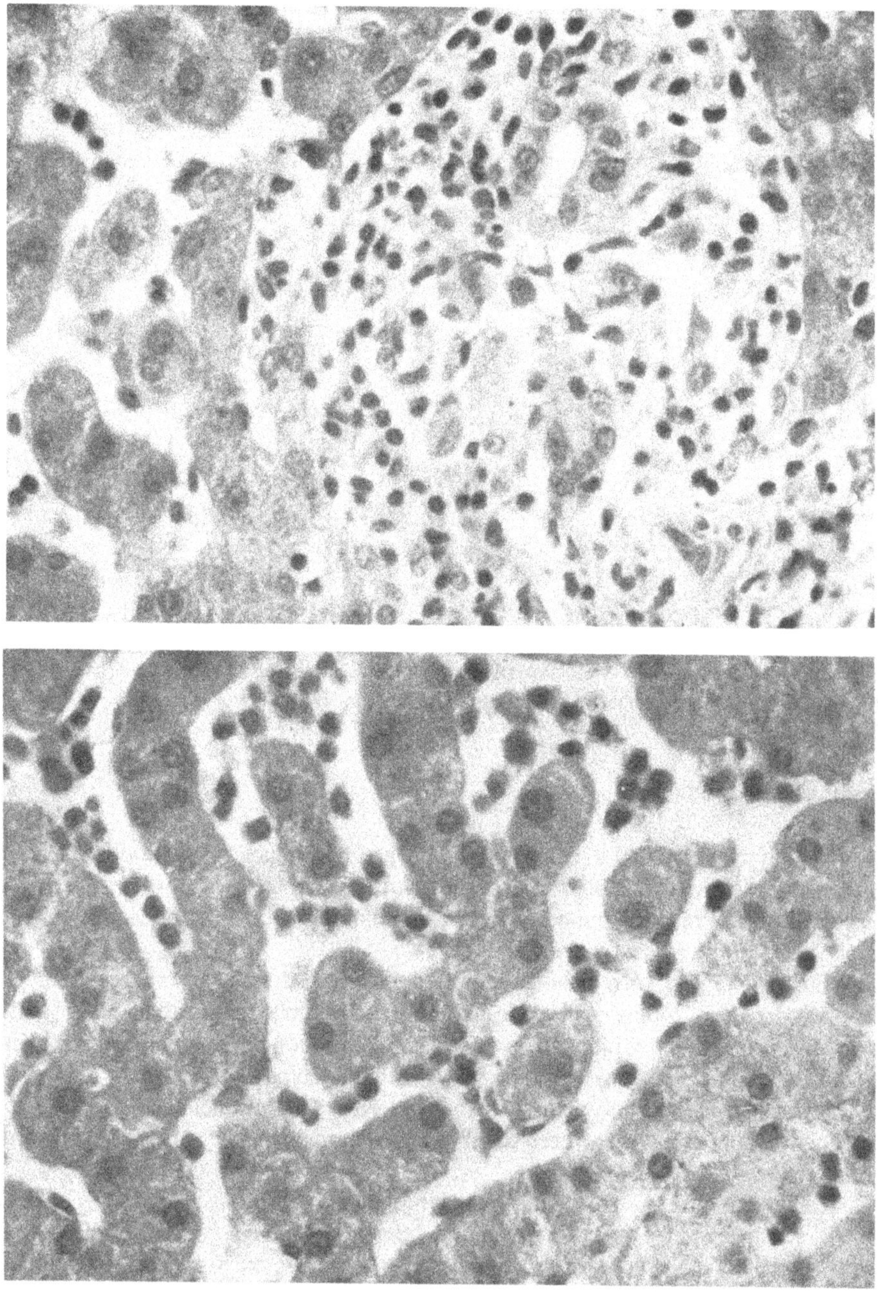

Fig. 3.8. Histology of the liver. H and E preparation

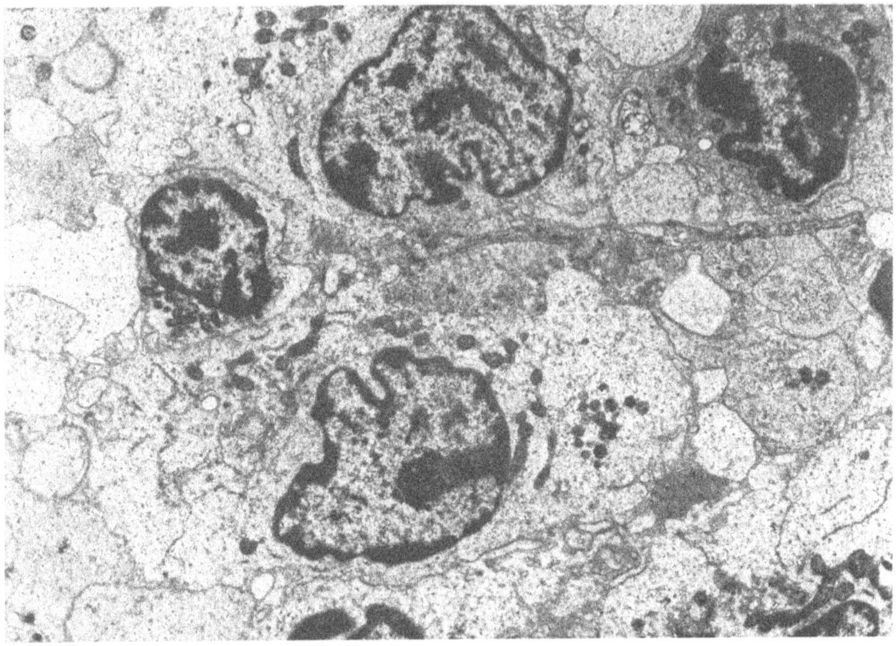

Fig. 3.9. Ultrastructure of a lymph node. There is clear HC infiltration of this node, but some of the normal architecture is preserved and at least one normal lymphocyte is seen (× 5,000)

3.4 Lymph Nodes

Although lymph-node enlargement in HCL is rarely prominent, when node material has been examined pathologically it has been shown to be involved in most instances [40]. Involved nodes are firm on macroscopic examination, and on sectioning they present a homogeneous white appearance.

Histologically, HC involvement is variable, sometimes seen as focal aggregations [202] and on other occasions as an extensive diffuse infiltration of most of the node [21, 40, 269]. However, even when massive infiltration is present, obliteration of the lymph node architecture is not total, and residual lymphocytes and lymphoid follicles are often seen (Fig. 3.9) [40, 70, 273]. Reticulin staining may show a normal pattern or a patchy increase in fibres [70]. Cells of fibroblastic appearance have been observed which may be responsible for the production of these reticulin fibres [269, 273].

Clinical infections may be associated with lymphadenopathy and, although HCs persist in the nodes, reactive changes are prominent and account for the increase in size. Plasma cells are particularly conspicuous in such nodes and can be shown to display polyclonal immunoglobulin staining [153].

4 The Hairy Cell: Cytological Aspects

4.1 Cytology

Hairy cells derive their name from the irregular fine cytoplasmic projections that extend for variable distances from the periphery. It is, in fact, a combination of characteristics that identifies the HC in ROMANOWSKY preparations: the eccentric nucleus with its fine chromatin condensation, the pale slate-blue cytoplasm, as well as the fine surface projections, all form part of the initial diagnostic impression (Figs. 4.1 and 4.2).

The mononuclear HC is larger than most lymphocytes, with a diameter of 15–30 μm and a modal cell volume by electronic measurement of approximately 450 μm^3 [33, 342]. In

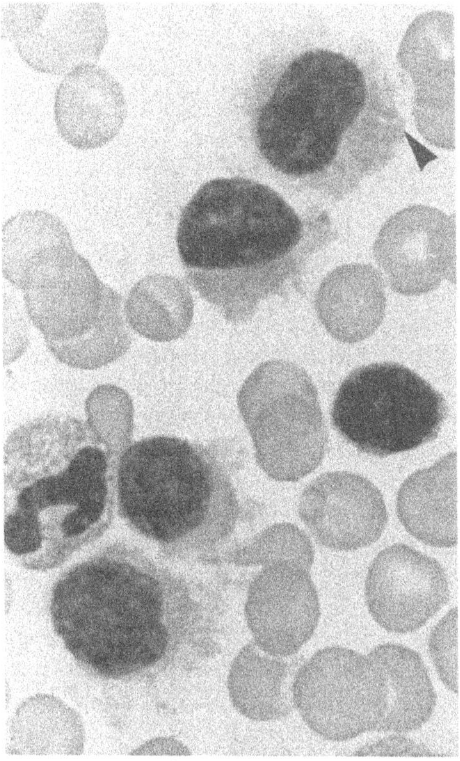

Fig. 4.1

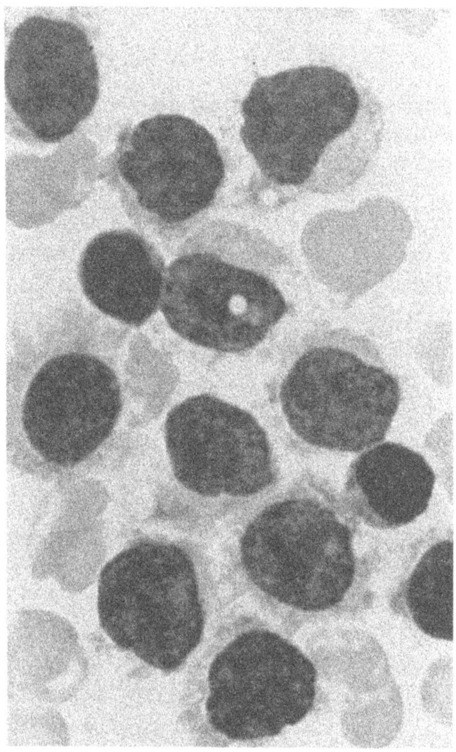

Fig. 4.2

Fig. 4.1. ROMANOWSKY preparation. In this buffy-coat preparation there are four typical HCs, a lymphocyte and a neutrophil. One of the HCs contains a cylindrical structure (▲); these inclusions were acid phosphatase-positive (Fig. 4.5)

Fig. 4.2. ROMANOWSKY preparation. This buffy-coat preparation containing eleven HCs and two lymphocytes demonstrates the range of nuclear morphology seen in HCL

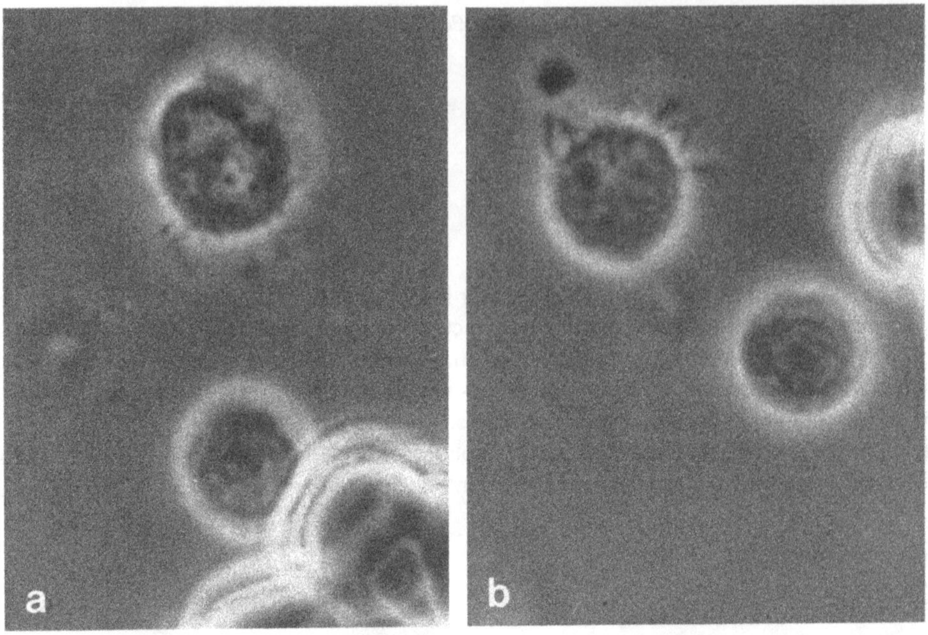

Fig. 4.3a, b. Phase-contrast preparation. The surface hairs of the HC are clearly seen. The nearby lymphocyte lacks surface projections. In the actively motile cell (**b**), the surface hairs are concentrated to one pole

ROMANOWSKY preparations the surface projections often produce no more than an ill-defined fringe to the cell outline: it is the frequency and fine nature of the hairs that distinguish them from the surface projections often seen in a variety of other cell types [354]. The surface hairs are more conspicuous in fresh wet preparations, especially under phase-contrast microscopy (Fig. 4.3), but are probably very much longer than is apparent in either ROMANOWSKY or phase preparations, since very long fine filaments can often be seen extending from cells stained with fluoresceinated anti-HC serum. However, in some patients surface hairs may be completely absent from a proportion, or even the majority, of recognizably pathological cells; these cells can be identified by their nuclear structure and cytoplasmic staining.

The nuclear : cytoplasmic ratio is generally intermediate between the high ratio of lymphocytes and many leukaemic blast cells and the low ratio of monocytes, macrophages, and some leukaemic monocyte precursors. The eccentrically placed nucleus is usually round or oval, there may be indentation or cleavage, and a folded or kidney shape may be seen. Moreover, the nuclear structure is less reticular than that of monocytes, with a mixture of finely dispersed and more coarsely clumped chromatin sometimes giving a checker-board or spongy appearance [29, 325, 339], while the occasional predominance of the finely dispersed pattern may recall the appearance of ground glass [373]. An overall dense, pachychromatic, nuclear staining, like that of the normal lymphocyte, is virtually never seen. Nucleoli are rarely conspicuous in ROMANOWSKY preparations, but small, usually single, nucleoli may be visible in a minority of hairy cells in smears stained with haematoxylin, as in counterstained PAS preparations (Fig. 4.4).

The cytoplasm stains a slate-blue colour with ROMANOWSKY stains, in which respect it is again intermediate between the sky-blue of the lymphocyte cytoplasm and the grey of the

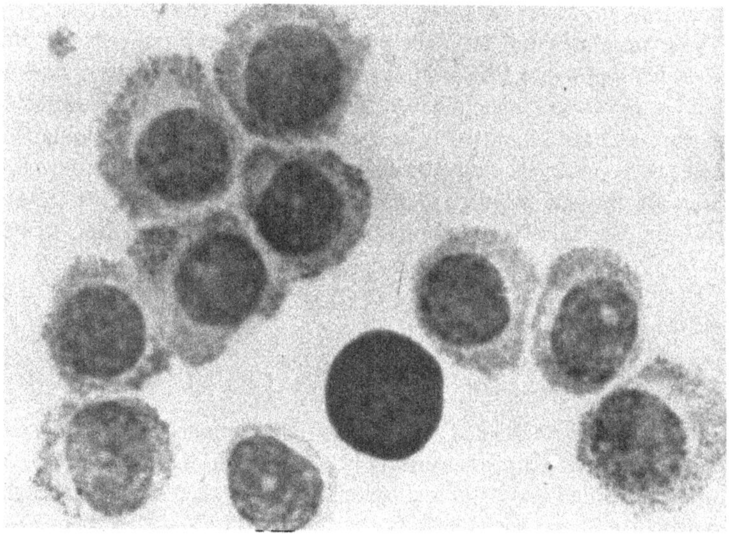

Fig. 4.4. PAS preparation. The HCs demonstrate variable patterns of PAS positivity, ranging from fine and diffuse to coarse and granular. The single granulocyte is strongly positive. The nucleoli of the HCs are evident in this preparation counterstained with haematoxylin

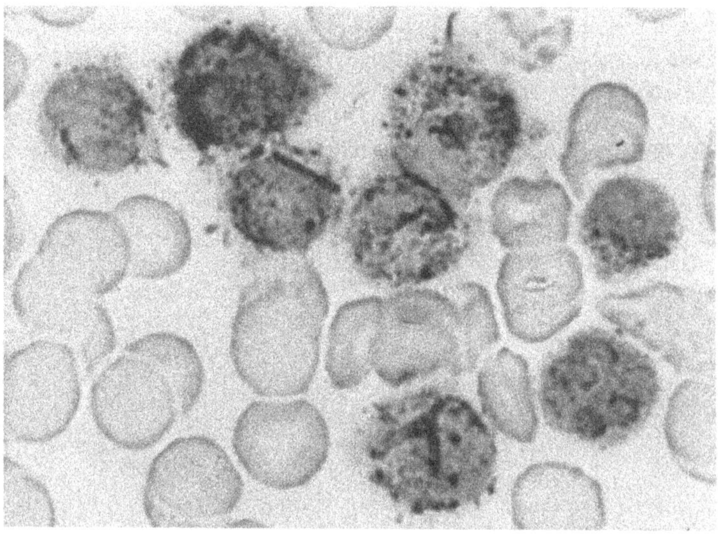

Fig. 4.5. Rod-shaped inclusions in HCs. Acid phosphatase preparation. All the HCs contain strong enzyme activity and the inclusions are clearly seen as positive rods

monocyte, and but less basophilic than the cytoplasm of most immature haemic cells. The structure sometimes appears homogeneous, but patchy variations in density are common and vacuoles are frequently seen. Despite reports to the contrary [28, 70], the cytoplasm may occasionally contain small azurophilic granules. Rod-shaped inclusions, negatively staining or with a negative core in a positively stained envelope, have been reported in ROMANOWSKY preparations and have been thought to represent R-L complexes (see Sect. 4.3.1) [125, 202, 208]. These structures may be made more conspicuous if the cells are first allowed to spread on glass before staining [93, 340]. We have only rarely seen distinct cylindrical structures of this kind in ROMANOWSKY-stained slides, but they are readily identified in toluidine blue-stained smears and semi-thin plastic sections. We have observed similar inclusions (Fig. 4.1) appearing as positively stained rods in acid-phosphatase preparations (Fig. 4.5) but have not been able to establish their identity, since electron microscope (EM) sections from material showing the light microscope inclusions did not reveal R-L complexes.

4.2 Cytochemistry

4.2.1 Acid Phosphatase

Seven isoenzymes of acid phosphatase are demonstrable in normal and pathological leucocytes by gel electrophoresis [235, 387]. The distribution of these isoenzymes among different normal and pathological cell types has been studied in detail by LI et al., who have shown that isoenzyme 5 is largely restricted to the HCs of HCL, in which it constitutes the major isoenzyme type [205, 223, 235, 267, 386]. This observation proved of great diagnostic significance, since it was demonstrated that isoenzyme 5, unlike the other acid-phosphatase enzymes (apart from isoenzyme 0 of Gaucher's disease), is resistant to L (+) tartrate [235] and can therefore be demonstrated by a simple cytochemical method [205, 387].
Consistent cytochemical demonstration of TRAP activity in HCs requires attention to several technical factors, which have been carefully reviewed by JANCKILA et al. [187, 188]. The different acid-phosphatase isoenzymes preferentially hydrolyse different substrates [224, 234], and naphthyl ASBI phosphoric acid is particularly suitable for the demonstration of isoenzyme 5 [188]. The sensitivity of this reaction is determined by the coupler used: fast garnet GBC produces maximum sensitivity and is recommended for the demonstration of TRAP

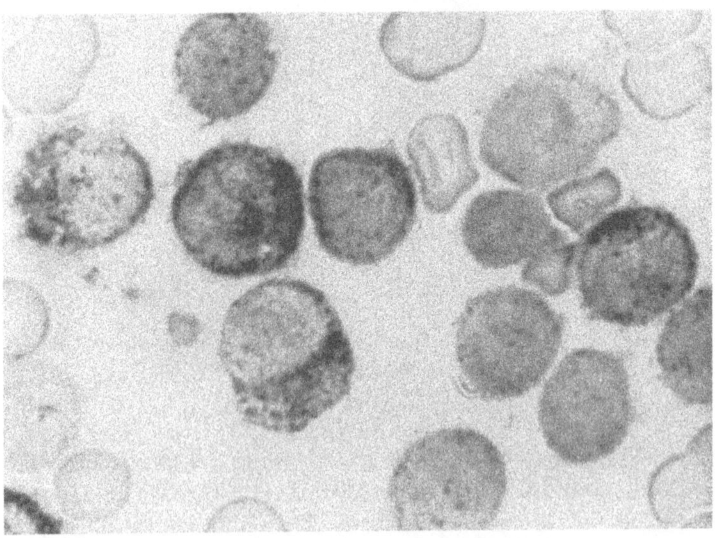

Fig. 4.6. TRAP preparation. Enzyme activity is seen in all the HCs, but ranges from strong and coarse to weak and finely scattered granular activity

in peripheral blood HCs [188]. Hexasotized pararosaniline as coupler is less sensitive and is therefore not optimal for peripheral blood smears, but the specific fine reaction product of the method makes it suitable for histological sections and dab preparations, where fast garnet GBC frequently gives nonspecific precipitates. To avoid errors attributable to enzyme inactivation, material should be incubated with and without tartrate, and tartrate-sensitive activity must be demonstrable in neutrophils.

A minority of cases of HCL may show little or no TRAP positivity [40, 63, 177, 185, 204, 332, 340], but at least some of the HCs from the great majority of reported cases have contained TRAP. It is not clear to what extent the few reported negative results are attributable to technical factors such as the use of pararosaniline, rather than fast garnet, as coupler [177, 204]. Certainly, in our series, all 27 patients studied by the naphthyl ASBI phosphate/fast garnet GBC method had a proportion of strongly TRAP-positive HCs. Most morphological HCs contained strong TRAP (Fig. 4.6), and a proportion of cells with lymphoid morphology (0%–40%) showed weaker scattered granular activity in many instances. Even in cases in which most morphological HCs disappeared from the peripheral blood (Sect. 2.6.2), occasional TRAP-positive cells could always be found.

4.2.2 Esterase

Hairy cells possess non-specific esterase (NSE) activity demonstrable with α-naphthyl butyrate, α-naphthyl acetate, or α-naphthyl ASD acetate as substrate, but lack chloroacetate esterase. (A single case of HCL with chloroacetate esterase activity has been described [276].)

Human leucocytes contain nine esterase isoenzymes, which show varying substrate specificity, and some of these have been associated with particular cell types [236]. It has not been determined whether HCs possess one specific isoenzyme type, but they show a distinctive pattern of NSE staining, consisting of a mixture of scattered fine granules, together with coarser granules sometimes localized in a crescentic configuration [177] (Fig. 4.7). With an

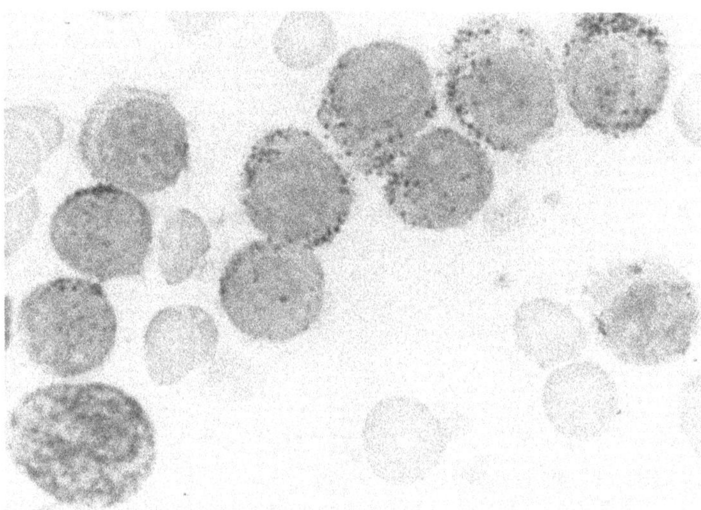

Fig. 4.7. NSE preparation. The HCs contain scattered granular positivity, which is sometimes localized in a crescentic configuration, even in some of the HCs with a more lymphoid morphology

α-naphthyl butyrate/fast garnet GBC method we have consistently been able to demonstrate this pattern in 20 cases of HCL. However, the NSE activity of HCs is never as strong as that commonly seen in monocytes, and many of the technical factors relevant for acid-phosphatase staining [188] probably affect the result [276]. We and others [32, 177, 335, 373] have found that the NSE of HCs (unlike that of monocytes) is not inhibited by fluoride, but the contrary view has been expressed [199]. As with the TRAP stain, we have regularly found that in addition to most morphological HCs, a proportion of cells with a lymphoid morphology display the pattern of NSE staining typical of HCs. Many of these lymphoid cells can be shown by immunological methods to be involved in the lymphoproliferation (Chap. 5).

4.2.3 Periodic Acid-Schiff (PAS)

Most HCs stain with the periodic acid-Schiff (PAS) method [70, 166, 254, 258, 286, 322, 373, 386]. The cells give weak or moderately strong diffuse staining, frequently with scattered fine, and sometimes coarse, stippling (Fig. 4.4).

4.2.4 β-Glucuronidase

HCs typically show scattered fine granules of positive staining for β-glucuronidase [276, 322, 386].

4.2.5 Other Cytochemical Methods

The following methods give either negative or minimal staining of HCs: adenosine deaminase, alkaline phosphatase, aminopeptidase, 5-nucleotidase, naphthylamidase, nitroblue tetrazolium reduction, Sudan black, oil red 0, toluidine blue and iron (Prussian blue) [64, 70, 218, 253, 276, 286, 322, 335, 372, 373, 386]. Peroxidase is also negative when staining is performed by standard methods on fixed cells [70, 276, 286, 322, 335, 373], but unfixed cells may contain weak peroxidatic activity under certain reaction conditions (see Sect. 4.3: Ultrastructure) [311, 312]. HCs are either negative or weakly positive for *N*-acetyl β-glucosaminidase [373, 386], and in methyl green pyronin stains show weak or absent pyroninophilia [335, 373] but positive staining of R-L complexes [125].
It has been conclusively shown by both biological [64, 70] and immunocytological methods that HCs lack lysozyme [297, 335].

4.2.6 Terminal Deoxynucleotidyl Transferase (TdT)

HCs contain variable, but usually low, amounts of biochemically detectable TdT activity [356]. The levels of enzyme expression are comparable with, or lower than, those of B-cell lines, and very much lower than the levels in thymus and ALL cells [356].

4.3 Ultrastructure

4.3.1 Transmission Electron Microscopy (TEM)

Numerous studies [5, 27, 42, 70, 93, 139, 140, 166, 186, 203, 206, 261, 284, 286, 322, 323, 357, 367, 372] have shown that at the ultrastructural level, as at the level of light microscopy, the HC displays a characteristic and distinctive appearance (Fig. 4.8). The fine-structural features are those of a metabolically active cell deriving much of its energy from oxidative mitochondrial metabolism.

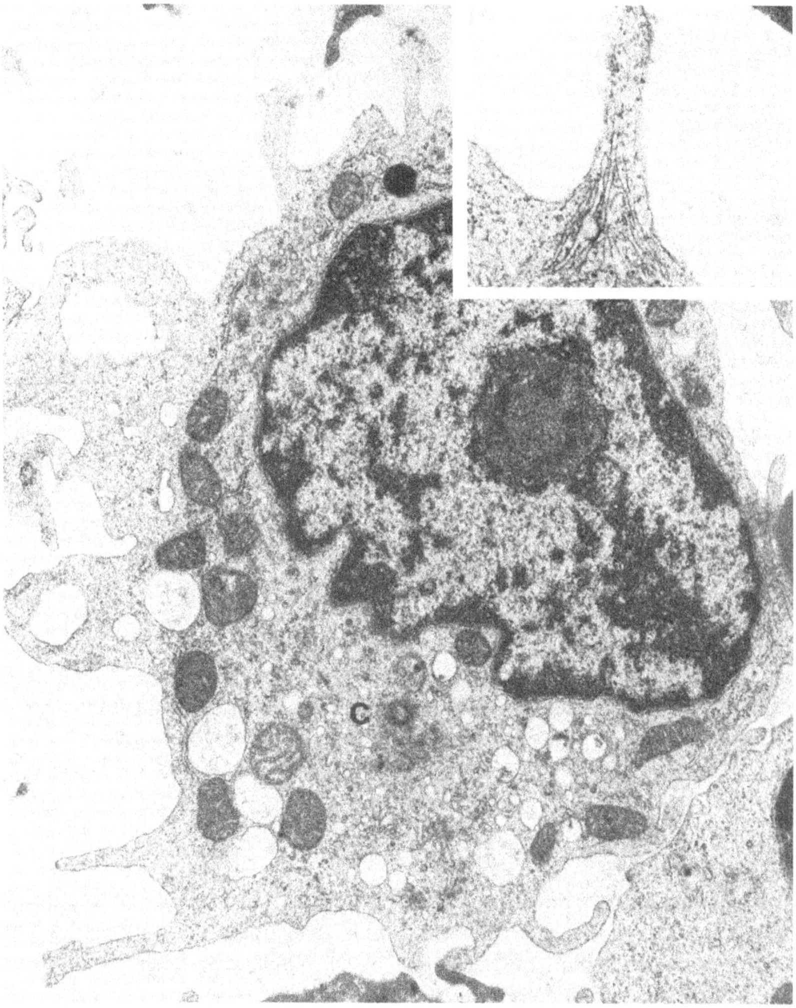

Fig. 4.8. Hairy cell. To minimize preparative artifact, this specimen was obtained by dextran sedimentation and fixation in suspension. Fine microvilli and more broadly based surface projections are present. The *inset* shows how microfibrils are seen entering the microvilli in favourable planes of section. Vacuoles and vesicles of varying size are particularly prominent in this cell. A centriole (*C*) is present in transverse section and microtubules are seen converging on the nearby pericentriolar satellites. The eccentric nuclear profile with its moderate peripheral chromatin condensation is typical; the nucleolus contains a distinct *pars amorpha* and a poorly defined nucleolonema (× 16,000; *inset* × 27,000)

Nucleus. The precise nuclear contour is dependent on the plane of section and on details of preparative technique (e.g., prolonged standing at room temperature before fixation may increase folding and indentation; Fig. 4.9), but there is variation from cell to cell and from case to case. The single nuclear profile usually seen often displays one or more indentations, and nuclear pockets are rare [203, 323]. Peripheral chromatin condensation is slight to moderate unless the heterochromatin is sectioned tangentially, when the condensation may appear

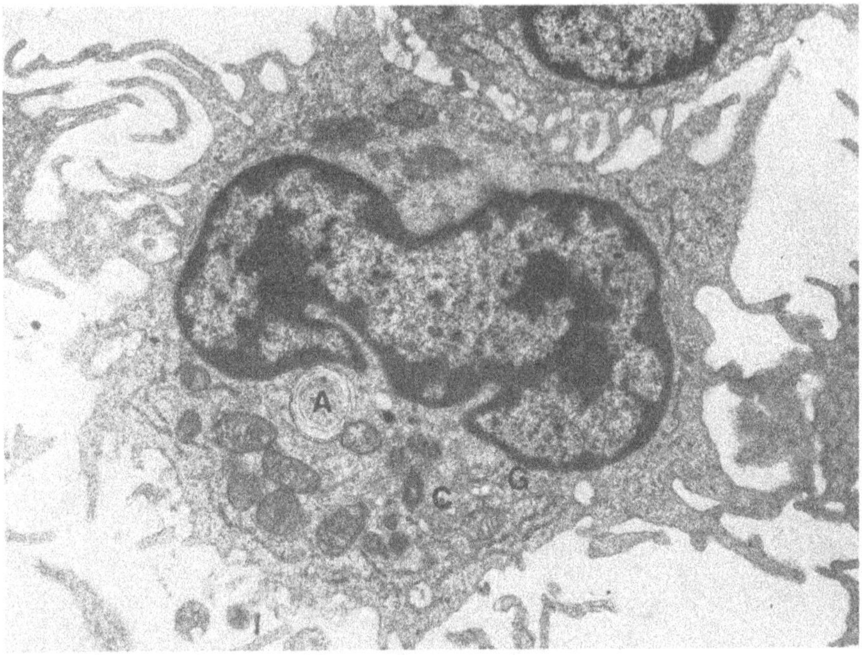

Fig. 4.9. Hairy cell. The "points" of the nuclear folds are directed towards the centriolar apparatus (*C*) of the cell. This appearance is particularly prominent when blood is allowed to stand for prolonged periods before fixation. A probable autophagic vacuole (*A*) is present; such structures may be surrounded by a rim of precipitate when acid-phosphatase cytochemistry is performed. A poorly developed Golgi-apparatus (*G*) is present (× 13,000)

conspicuous. Many nuclear profiles lack nucleoli, but when these structures are present they are nearly always single and are not highly developed; only occasionally are distinct *pars amorpha* and nucleolonema seen (Fig. 4.10). Nuclear bodies may occasionally be present (Fig. 4.10) but are uncommon.

Cytoplasm. As with the nucleus, the precise appearance of the cytoplasm is somewhat variable, depending not only on the particular case under study but also on the plane of section and on preparative technique. For example, when phosphate, rather than cacodylate, is used to buffer the glutaraldehyde fixative, the cytoplasm takes on a more dense appearance and the organelles are less readily identified. However, the surface projections of HCs are a consistent feature and are not critically dependent on optimal fixation, being well seen even after harsh handling, imperfect fixation, and preservation with fixatives of widely different osmolarity. The surface projections are of two main types [203]: numerous fine microvilli and less frequent broadly based structures (Fig. 4.8) (see Sect. 4.3.2). In favourable sections (Fig. 4.8, inset), large numbers of microfilaments can be seen entering the microvilli, and these are presumably concerned with their structural stability. Centrifugation before fixation is said to result in apparent lengthening of microvilli and in the formation of small blebs both at the cell surface and within the microvilli [203]. In most cases, occasional otherwise typical HCs are seen to lack surface projections, and in a few patients such cells are prominent, even when great care is taken with fixation.

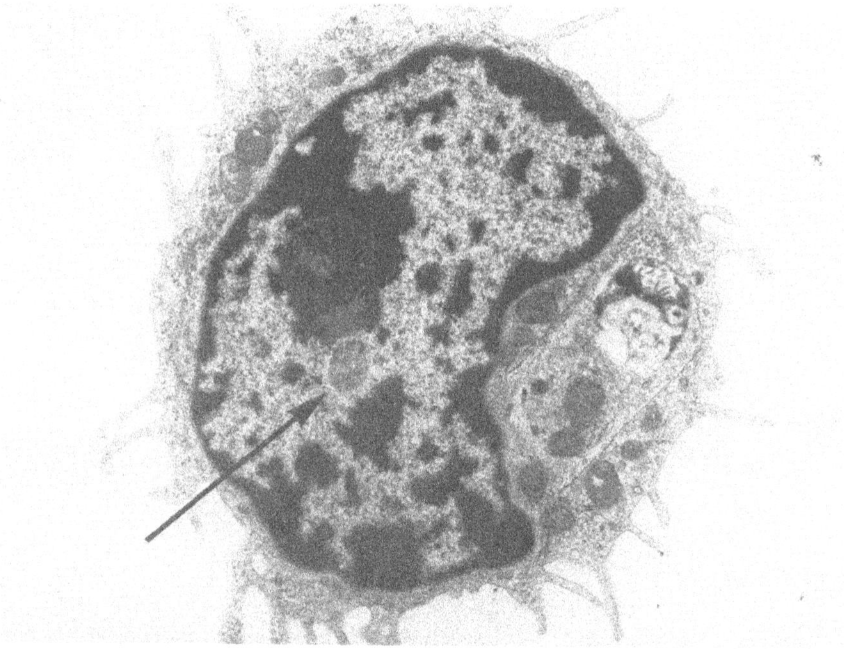

Fig. 4.10. Hairy cell. The nucleus contains an especially well-developed nucleolus with distinct *pars amorpha* and nucleolonema. A probable nuclear body (*arrow*) lies close to the nucleolus. Two autophagic vacuoles are present; the contents of the upper one are at a later stage of digestion (× 13,000)

The cytoplasm frequently contains numerous vacuoles and vesicles (Fig. 4.8) of variable size and shape. Many of the larger vacuoles are probably pinocytotic vacuoles formed by coalescence of neighbouring surface folds, while the smaller vesicles may represent micropinocytosis resulting from invagination of the surface membrane. Some vacuoles contain altered cytoplasmic material and are readily identified as autophagic vacuoles (Figs. 4.9 and 4.10); in others (Fig. 4.11) the material is so altered that it is not possible to determine whether the vacuole is autophagic or phagocytic. Very occasionally, an internalized erythrocyte may be seen [93] (Fig. 4.12). We have not observed thrombophagocytosis, but this has been described [322].

In many planes of section, the cytoplasm appears agranular, but in others a number of membrane-bound granular structures of varying size and shape may be seen (Figs. 4.12 and 4.13). The most frequent granule type is small and displays an electron-dense core surrounded by a peripheral pale zone (Figs. 4.12 and 4.13). Occasional larger dense granules, sometimes with an ill-defined membranous content, may be seen. At least some of both types of granules can be shown to possess acid-phosphatase activity and therefore to be lysosomes. An increase in granules has been noted after short-term culture [286]. Lipid droplets (Figs. 4.15 and 4.17) are frequent, but are readily distinguished from the granules by the absence of a limiting membrane, their larger size, and their weak staining pattern.

In suitably stained material, the HC can frequently be seen to contain significant amounts of glycogen, which is either scattered diffusely through the cytoplasm as single granules or, sometimes, arranged as small collections of particles (Fig. 4.14); this distribution of glycogen

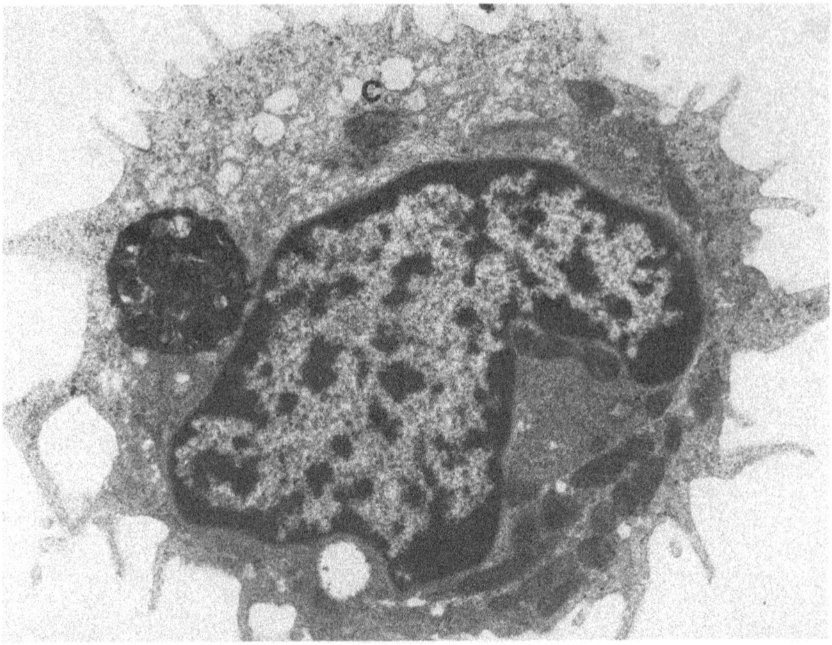

Fig. 4.11. Hairy cell. The contents of the dense membrane-bound structure are so altered that it is not possible to determine whether it is an autophagic or a phagocytic vacuole. Five transversely sectioned R-L complexes are present, and the centriolar apparatus (*C*) with associated microtubules is prominent (× 14,500)

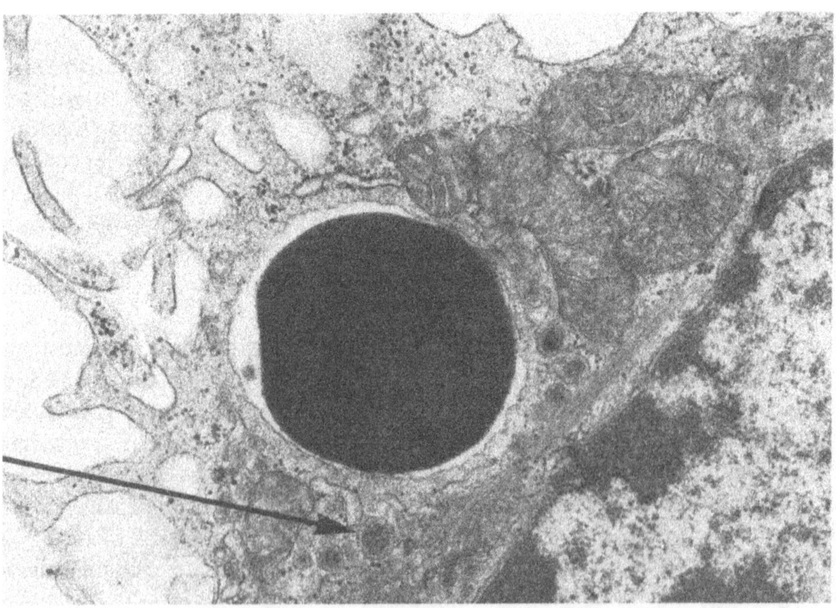

Fig. 4.12. Erythrophagocytosis by an HC. A spontaneously internalized erythrocyte is clearly seen. Several granules (*arrow*) with a peripheral clear zone are present nearby. In favourable sections these granules can be seen fusing with phagocytosed material (× 35,000)

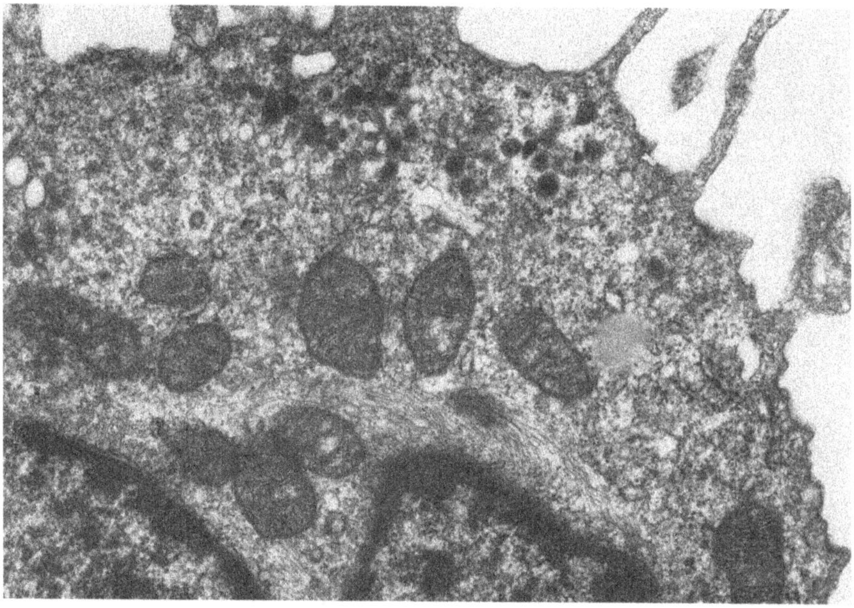

Fig. 4.13. Cytoplasmic granules in an HC. The granules are unusually prominent in this cell; many are seen to be made up of a central dense core surrounded by a peripheral pale zone. Longitudinally and transversely sectioned perinuclear fibrils are seen (× 26,500)

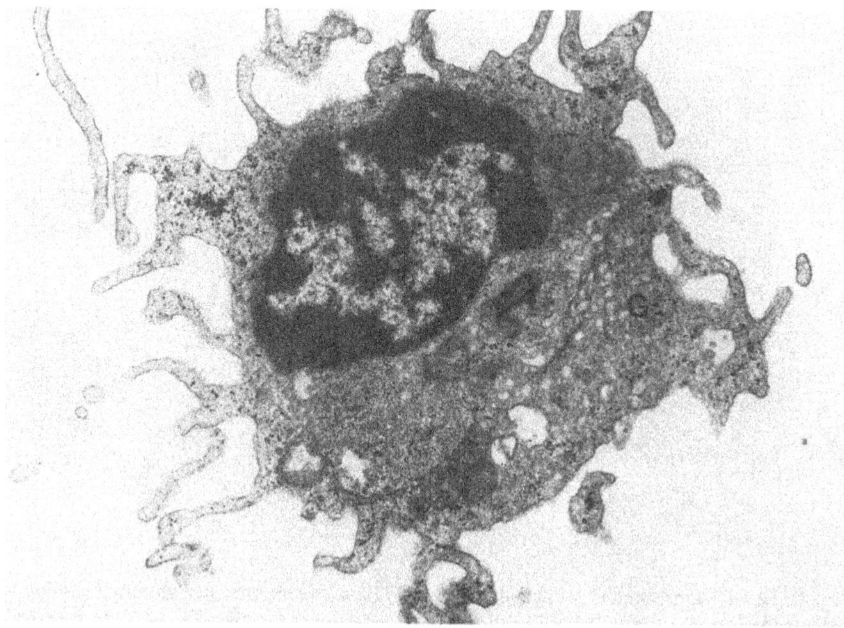

Fig. 4.14. Hairy cell. The glycogen is particularly well demonstrated in this cell and is seen scattered both as single granules and as small accumulations. Two R-L complexes are present. The Golgi apparatus (*G*) is better developed than in many HCs and a prominent centriole is seen. Lead citrate staining (× 12,000)

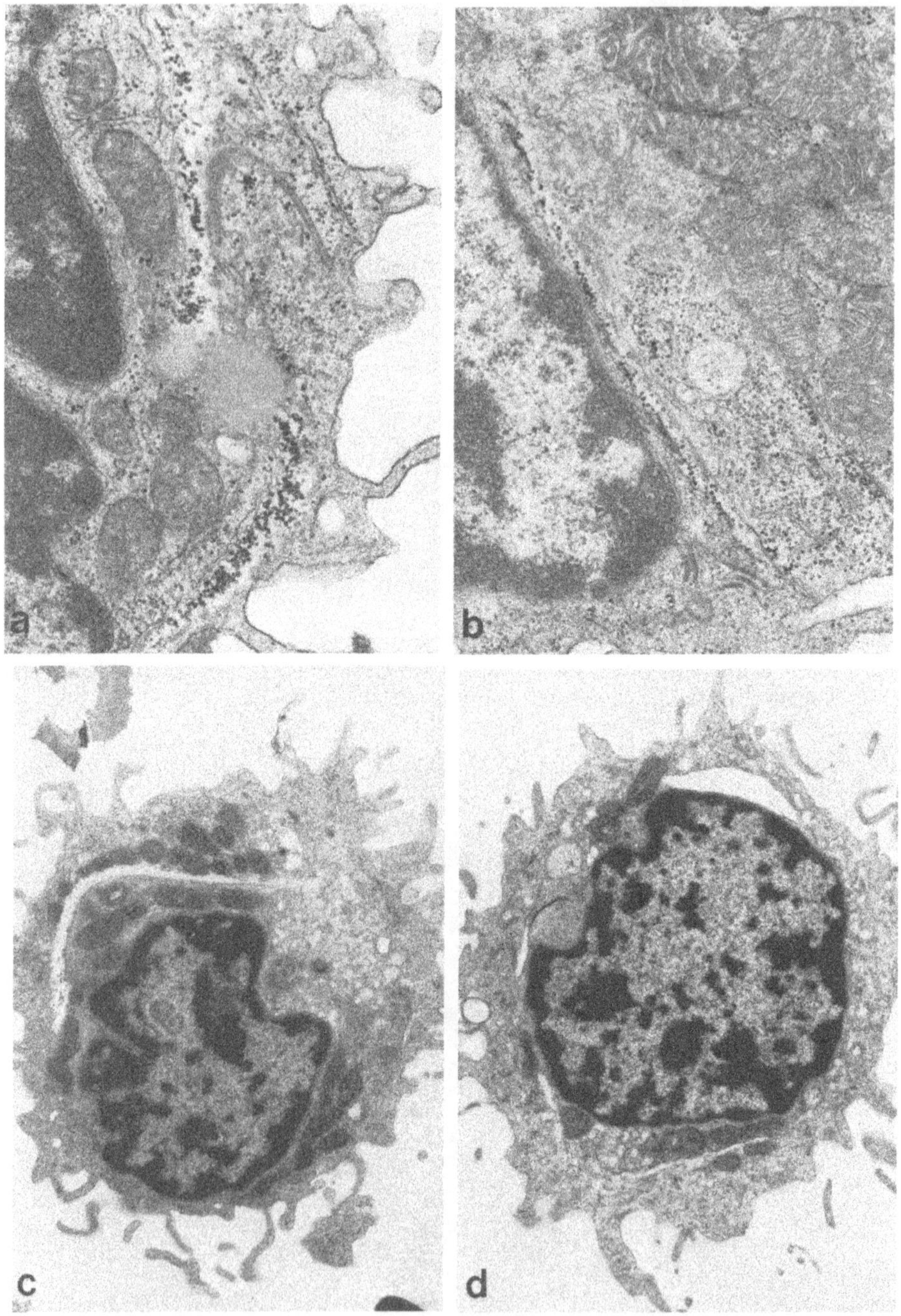

Fig. 4.15a–d. Membrane-glycogen structures in HCs. The membranes are often slightly wavy and arranged (**a**) in a crescentic configuration or (**b**) approximately linearly. The glycogen is frequently partially (**c**) or completely (**d**) extracted. Two lipids droplets are seen in **a** (**a** × 21,000; **b** × 27,000; **c** × 9,000; **d** × 9,000)

accounts for the diffuse and the fine granular PAS positivity of HCs (Sect. 4.2.3). In addition, the glycogen is sometimes associated with membranes to form the structures illustrated in Fig. 4.15. These structures, which have not been recorded in HCL by previous observers, are a constant and frequent feature of HCs, but their nature is not clear.

HCs contain abundant mitochondria with well-defined cristae that very occasionally contain cross-hatched structures [203] (Fig. 4.23). Modest numbers of monoribosomes and infrequent polyribosomes are scattered throughout the cytoplasm. A few short strands of rough endoplasmic reticulum (RER) are typically present, and these are frequently associated with any R-L complexes present (see below). Scattered agranular endoplasmic reticulum may also be observed in some sections.

The Golgi apparatus is only moderately developed, consisting of some three to five cisternae and a variable number of associated vesicles and vacuoles (Figs. 4.9 and 4.14). Prominent centrioles are frequently seen in the Golgi area, and microtubules, which extend throughout the cytoplasm of HCs, can often be observed converging on the conspicuous pericentriolar satellites (Figs. 4.8, 4.9, and 4.24). As in other cell types with nuclear clefts [73], microtubules are often prominent within the nuclear indentations of HCs and are probably involved in their formation.

Randomly orientated fibrils are also frequently prominent, especially in the perinuclear area of the cytoplasm.

Freeze-Etching. The freeze-etch technique, which avoids many of the artifacts produced by processing for the preparation of thin sections, has confirmed many of the ultrastructural features outlined above; in particular, similar distinctive surface projections are seen [42]. In addition, this technique has demonstrated a high density of nuclear pores and a monogranular distribution of intramembranous particles in HCs [42].

Ribosome-Lamella (R-L) Complexes. Ribosome-lamella complexes are distinctive structures (Figs. 4.11, 4.14, 4.16–4.18), which have been referred to by a number of other terms, including granulolamellar structures [93], tubular cytoplasmic inclusions [93], and lamellar bodies [217]. They were first described in HCs by Katayama et al. [206]. Although R-L complexes may occasionally be observed in a variety of other haematological [7, 37, 78, 217, 252, 357, 360, 383, 396] and nonhaematological [180, 268, 281, 368] cell types, they are more common in HCL than in other haematological malignancies [203], and are therefore of diagnostic significance. The function of R-L complexes is unknown, but they do not appear to be involved in immunoglobulin synthesis, since we have observed unstained rod-shaped inclusions in cells showing diffuse fluorescence with anti-immunoglobulin reagents.

Ribosome-lamella complexes have been reported to occur in approximately 50% of cases of HCL [63, 93, 125, 203] and in from 0.2% to almost 100% of the cells of a given case [93, 203]. We have observed R-L complexes in 14 of 23 cases and in 0–25% of individual peripheral blood mononuclear cells (mean 2%). The frequency of R-L complexes within a given case varies on different occasions of study, but if present in blood HCs they are also to be found in splenic cells (range 0%–18% of mononuclear cells; mean 2%).

As their name suggests, R-L complexes are composed of ribosomal granules associated with an elaborate system of fibrils (the lamellar component).

The granules of the complex measure approximately 200 Å in diameter and are identical with the monoribosomes in the neighbouring cytoplasm. Their RNA content has been confirmed by digestion with RNase [7, 38], by the demonstration of persistent electron density after the regressive staining procedure of Bernhard, and by the pyroninophilia of the complex at the level of light microscopy [93].

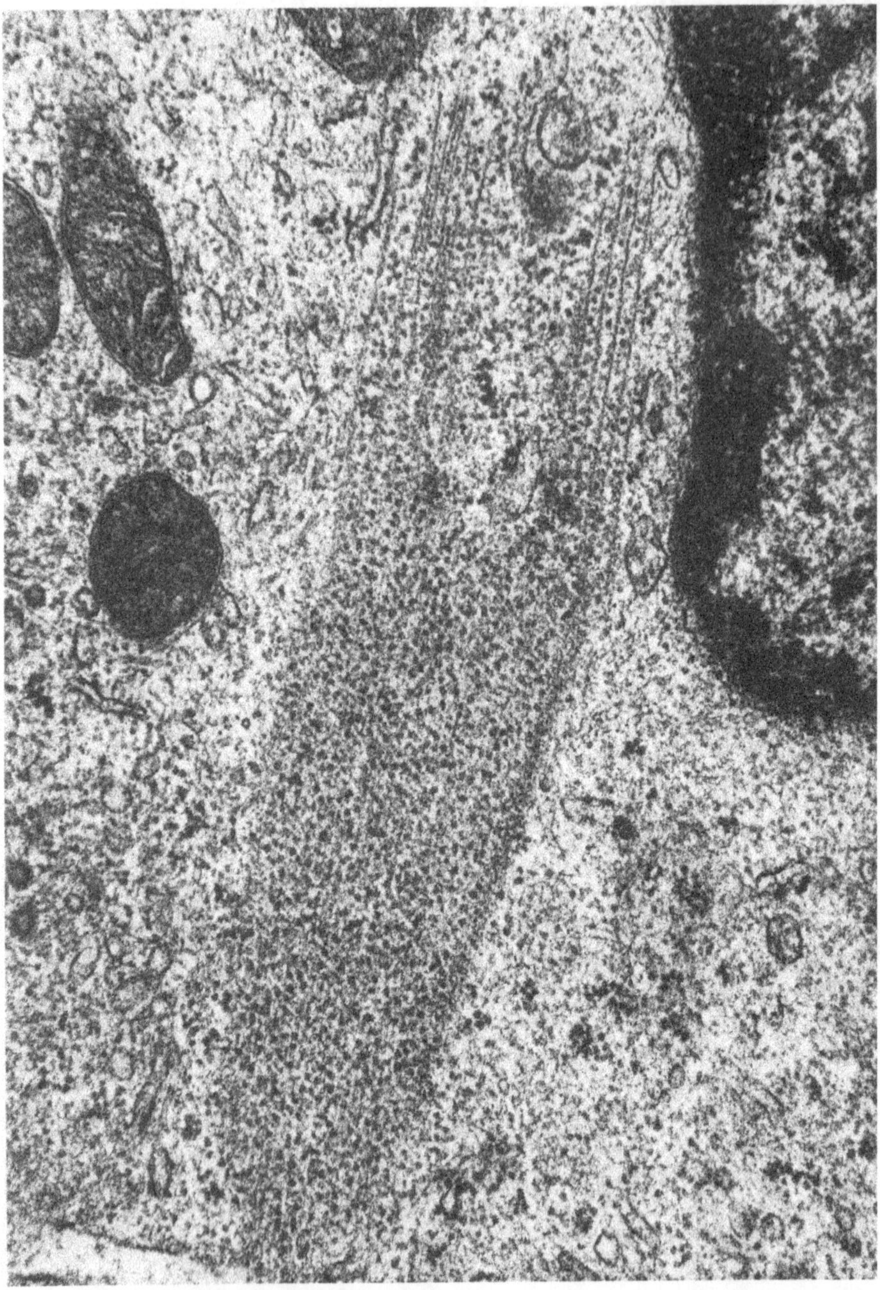

Fig. 4.16. R-L complex. In its upper part, the complex is sectioned longitudinally, but its lower part is cut obliquely. Careful examination of the obliquely sectioned area reveals the two-dimensional net-like structure described in the text (× 67,000)

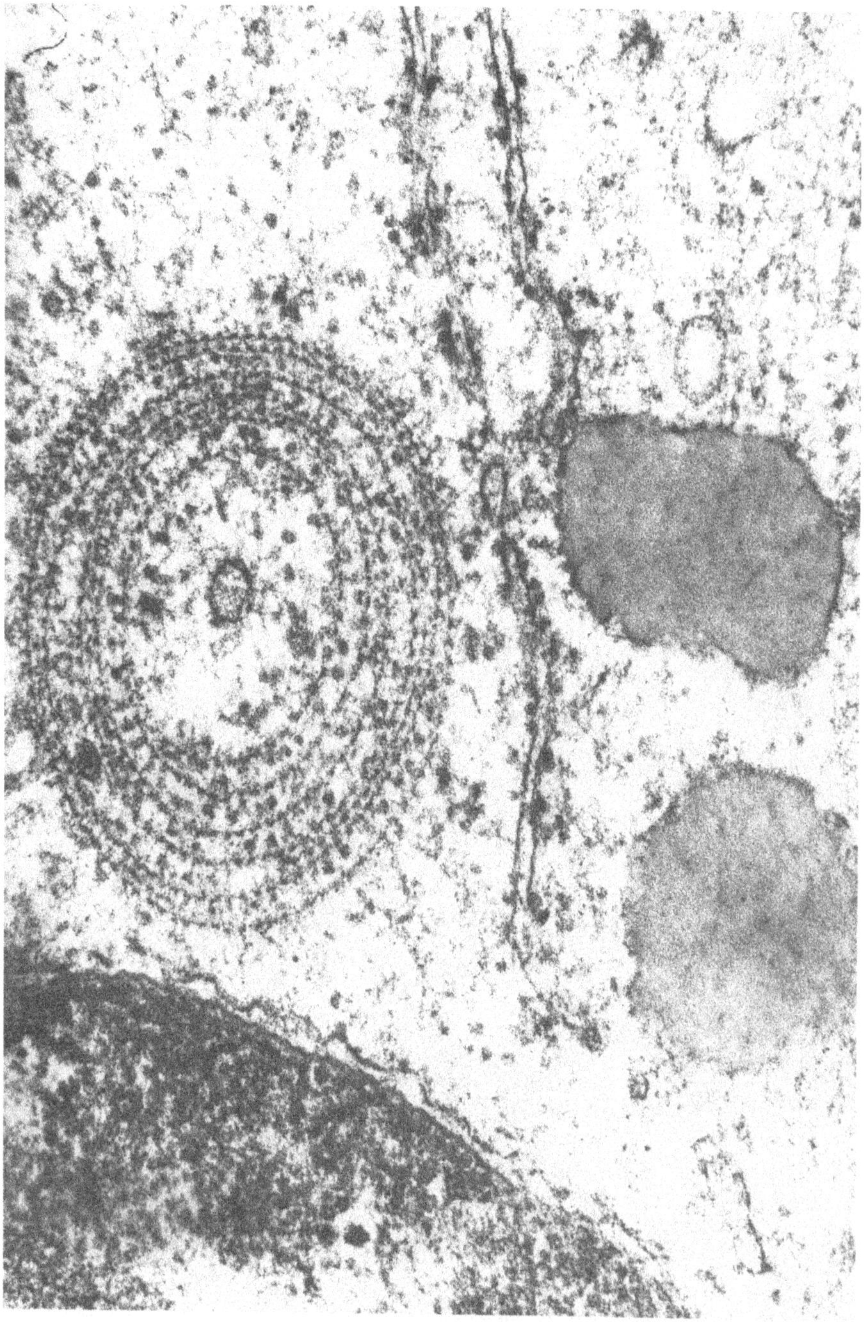

Fig. 4.17. R-L complex in transverse section. The coils of the lamellar component of the complex are seen to be composed of distinct subunits, which sometimes appear to be separated but are often joined. The ribosomes, which are concentrically arranged approximately midway between the coils, sometimes appear to be connected with the subunits of the lamellar component. Two prominent lipid droplets are present (× 90,000)

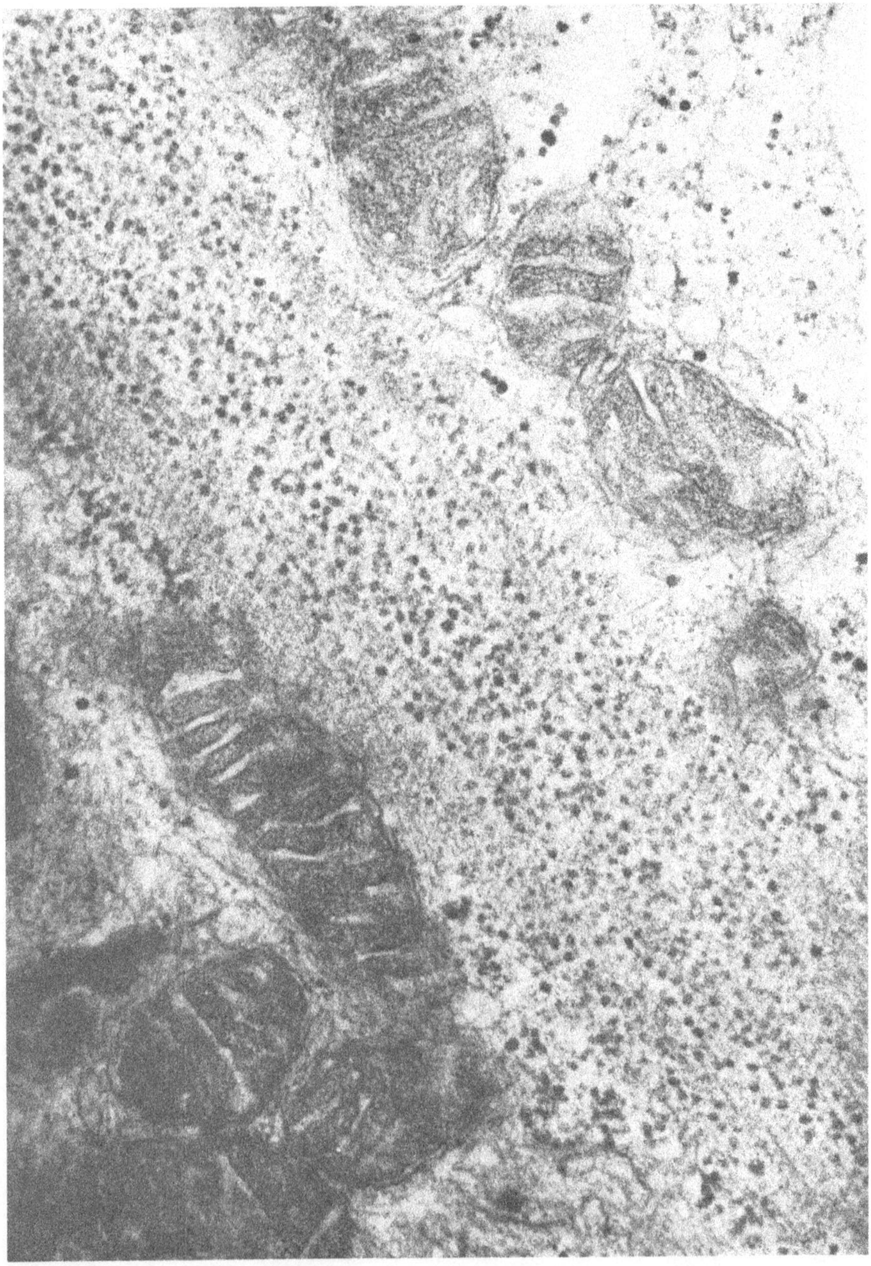

Fig. 4.18. R-L complex in oblique section. The net-like structure of the lamella component is clearly seen, particularly at each end of the complex (× 80,000)

The detailed structure of the lamellar component and its precise relationship to the ribosomes that form an integral part of the inclusion are complex and not fully known. However, the following details are clear. The basic profile of the complex differs from one section to another and may appear as parallel lines, concentric circles, or ellipsoids. In most planes of section, however, the R-L complexes are seen to possess a central core of cytoplasm approximately 400 nm wide (Figs. 4.16 and 4.17). In longitudinal section, the lamellar component is seen as multiple (up to eight) parallel straight fibres arranged on each side of the central core (Fig. 4.16). These fibrils of approximately 60–90 Å in diameter are usually regularly spaced some 450 Å apart and can sometimes be seen to be continuous with the less regularly arranged fibrils that extend throughout the cytoplasm of HCs [357]. The spaces between fibrils are occupied by parallel rows of ribosomes. The spacing of the ribosomes varies somewhat, but is usually 220–350 Å.

In transverse section, the central core is slightly oval in outline and the lamellar component appears as a two-dimensional coiled structure, while the ribosomes are arranged concentrically between the coils [93] (Fig. 4.17). At high power the coiled lamellae are seen to be composed of subunits (approx. 150 Å in diameter), which sometimes appear separated in the form of a dotted line, but often seem to be joined to give the appearance of a line with localized expansions (Fig. 4.17). It has been suggested that these subunits represent transverse sections of the parallel fibrils seen in longitudinal section [93].

The ultrastructural observations outlined above led Daniel and Flandrin [93] to propose that R-L complexes are hollow, cylindrical, coiled structures in which the coils are made up of rows of fibrils orientated parallel to the axis of the cylinder.

However, this model cannot be wholly correct, since we have repeatedly observed that in certain planes of section the lamellar component is not simply composed of parallel fibrils, but appears rather as a net-like structure comprising rows of finer pairs of fibrils arranged approximately at right angles to each other (Figs. 4.16 and 4.18). The gap between successive pairs of fibrils is of the order of 150 Å (Fig. 4.18). Although the ribosomes frequently do not appear to be attached to the lamellar component, in transverse sections rather ill-defined material can sometimes be seen connecting the ribosomes with the sectioned subunits of the lamellar component of the complex (Fig. 4.17). Perhaps, then, the coils in the model proposed by Daniel and Flandrin [93] are composed of a two-dimensional net of fibrils (Fig. 4.19) from which the ribosomes are suspended.

Ribosome-lamella complexes are sometimes closely associated with strands of RER. This association is most frequently observed at the outer surface of the complex (Fig. 4.16), but many also occur at the inner surface adjoining the central core. In longitudinal section, the strands of RER often run parallel with the longitudinal fibres of the complex, while in transverse section

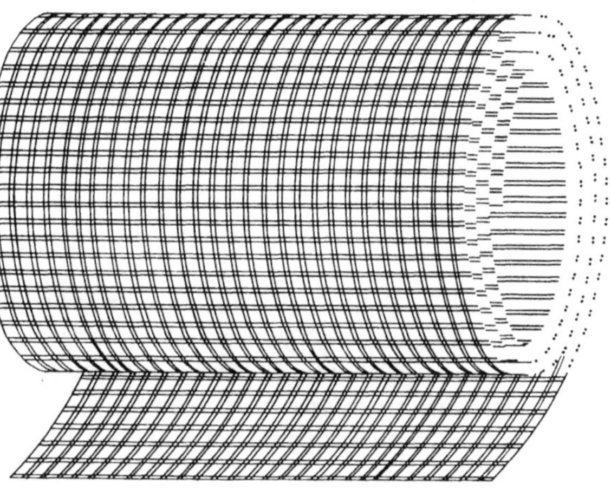

Fig. 4.19. The three-dimensional structure of the R-L complex. The model originally proposed by Daniel and Flandrin [93] is modified to take account of the net-like appearance of the lamellar component of the complex in certain planes of section

the strands appear curved, as if to follow the coiled lamellar component of the complex. This appearance has led DANIEL and FLANDRIN [93] to propose that the cylindrical R-L complex is partially ensheathed by a continuous sac of RER. The close association between R-L complexes and RER has also led to suggestions [37, 63] that RER is the fundamental structure of origin of the complex. Following up this suggestion, it has been proposed that the rounded profiles of RER sometimes seen in HCs represent an initial stage in the formation of the complex [37, 63]. However, it should be pointed out that numerous R-L complexes are frequently seen without associated RER. Again, we have only very occasionally observed rounded profiles of RER in HCs, even in cases with numerous R-L complexes. It therefore seems best to conclude that the origin of the R-L complex remains unknown.

Fibrillary Inclusions. We have frequently observed the type of fibrillary structure illustrated in Figs. 4.20–4.22. This inclusion, which does not seem to have been previously reported in HCL, was present in < 1%–15% (mean 2.5%) of the peripheral blood mononuclear cells in 15 of 23 cases of HCL examined. We did not, however, observe the structure in any of the 14 spleens examined. These inclusions measure up to 5 μm in length and 0.5 μm in width, and are composed of parallel arrays of fibrils (approx. 90 Å in diameter and some 100 Å apart) (Figs. 4.20–4.22), which can sometimes be seen to be continuous with the less regularly arranged fibrils of the cytoplasm. The three-dimensional appearance of these fibrillary structures is not clear, for we have not identified them with certainty in transverse section. Nevertheless, they may be bundles of fibrils, since localized collections of transversely sectioned fibrils (Fig. 4.20, inset) are frequently seen in cells in which the distinctive longitudinal structures are numerous. In many views, a regular transverse pattern of fibrils of similar dimensions to the more conspicuous longitudinal ones can also be observed (Fig. 4.22). In addition, broad, ill-defined darker zones can often be seen running transversely across the inclusion; these zones sometimes give the impression of irregular transverse banding (Fig. 4.21). Moreover, at high magnifications, both longitudinal and transverse fibres can be seen to be composed of two narrower parallel fibrils. Thus, the substructure of these inclusions resembles the net-like appearance observed in certain planes of section of the lamellar component of R-L complexes. This raises the possibility that the fibrillary structures are related to R-L complexes and might conceivably represent an uncoiled form of the lamellar component of the complex. However, they are not associated with ribosomes, they do not present intermediate stages of layering or coiling on longitudinal or transverse section, and they are frequently observed in cases in which no typical R-L complexes can be found. (Of 23 cases, six had fibrillary structures only, five had R-L complexes only, nine had both inclusions, and three had neither inclusion.) Whatever the nature of these structures, they are a characteristic feature of HCL. We have observed them in 65% of cases of the disease, but in none of the ten cases of CLL in which they were specifically looked for, despite the fact that R-L complexes were observed in one of these cases. Moreover, the distinctive closely spaced linear nature of the fibrillary structures of HCs is different from that of the wavy and more widely spaced bundles of fibrils commonly observed in normal and leukaemic monocytes [73].

Other Inclusions. Figure 4.23 illustrates a number of other types of inclusion occasionally seen in HCs. These have not been previously described in HCL, but we are unable to comment on their nature or significance, except that they are associated with endoplasmic reticulum. Tubuloreticular structures of a kind seen in a number of cell types have been described in HCs [374]. We have not observed such structures in HCs, although we have seen them in a variety of other types of leukaemic cell [74].

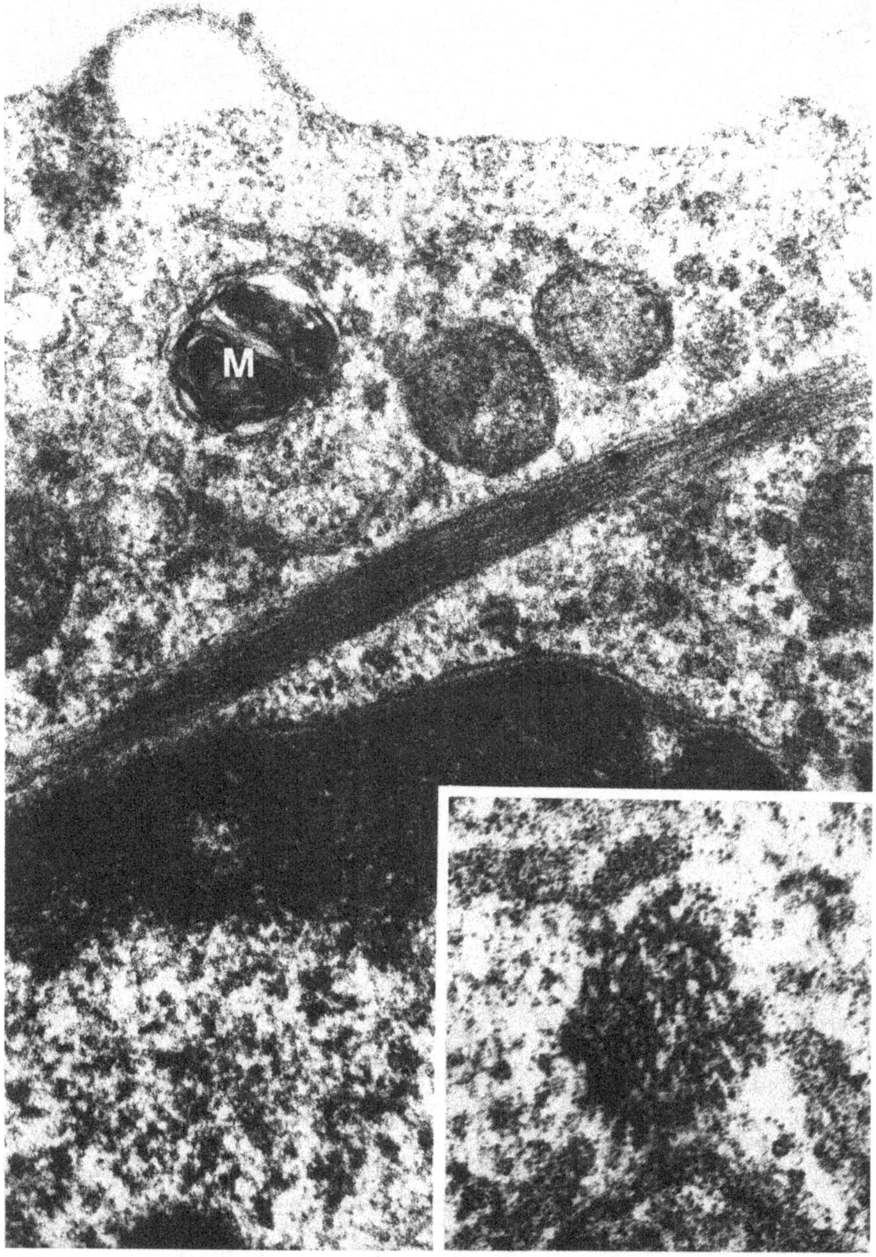

Fig. 4.20. Fibrillary inclusion. Needle-shaped inclusions of this type are frequently seen in HCs; similar, but broader, structures (Figs. 4.21 and 4.22) are less numerous, but not rare. The inclusion is seen to be composed of parallel fibrils. A myelin figure (*M*) is present (× 55,000). The *inset* shows the possible structure of the inclusion in transverse section (× 130,000)

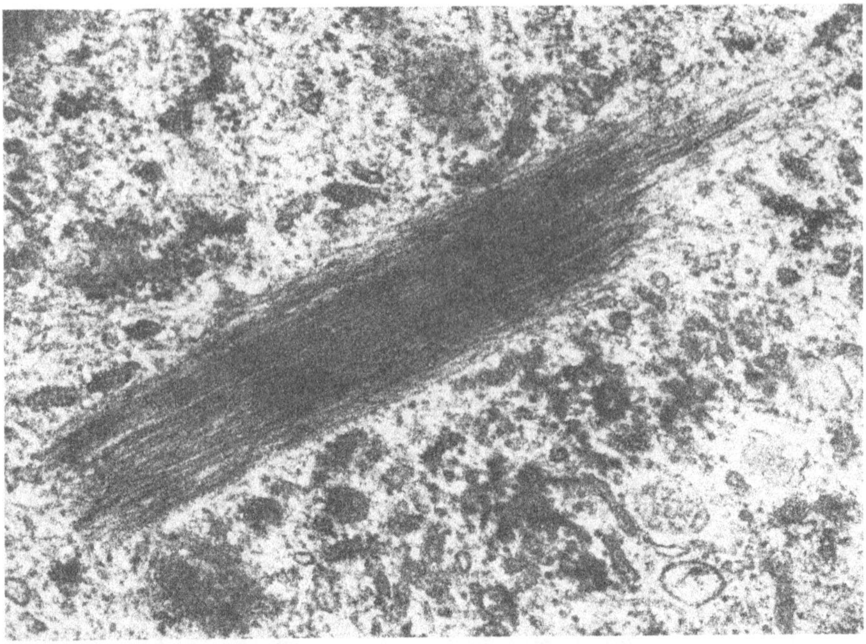

Fig. 4.21. Fibrillary inclusion. The inclusion is seen to be composed of parallel arrays of fibrils (approximately 90 Å diameter and 100 Å apart), and these appear to be continuous with less regularly arranged cytoplasmic fibrils. At least two broad ill-defined darker zones are visible running transversely across the inclusion. Scattered strands of rough and smooth endoplasmic reticulum are unusually prominent in this cell (× 47,000)

Zipper-like Junctions or Langerhans-like Granules. These distinctive surface structures have been described in HCs by a number of authors [17, 93, 283, 373], but may also be found in a variety of other haematological proliferations, including both monocytic [329] and lymphoid [203] cell types. The term Langerhans-like granules is derived from the fact that similar structures are observed in epidermal Langerhans cells.

The zipper-like junctions display a pentalaminar structure with a central lamella midway between two lateral limiting membranes, each of which displays a double outline at high power (Fig. 4.24). The structures are usually located at or near the cell surface and may be observed between adjacent cells or between interacting membranes of the same cell. Their surface nature has been confirmed by the observation of ruthenium-red staining of the space on either side of the central lamella [284]. Zipper-like junctions are only very rarely seen in HCs [93, 203], but an increased frequency after phagocytosis, particularly of bacteria, has been reported [93]. We have not observed this increase after phagocytosis of latex particles. Nor can we confirm any association between the zipper-like junctions and skin involvement [17, 284], since we have observed them in patients without any dermatological abnormality.

Ultrastructural Cytochemistry. Acid phosphatase has been demonstrated in some, but usually not all, the cytoplasmic granules of HCs (Fig. 4.25) and in occasional strands of RER [5, 44, 101, 207, 322]. After HCs have been incubated with latex particles, acid phosphatase-positive granules can occasionally be observed fusing with the membrane surrounding internalized latex particles, and a proportion of the particles are coated with enzyme activity

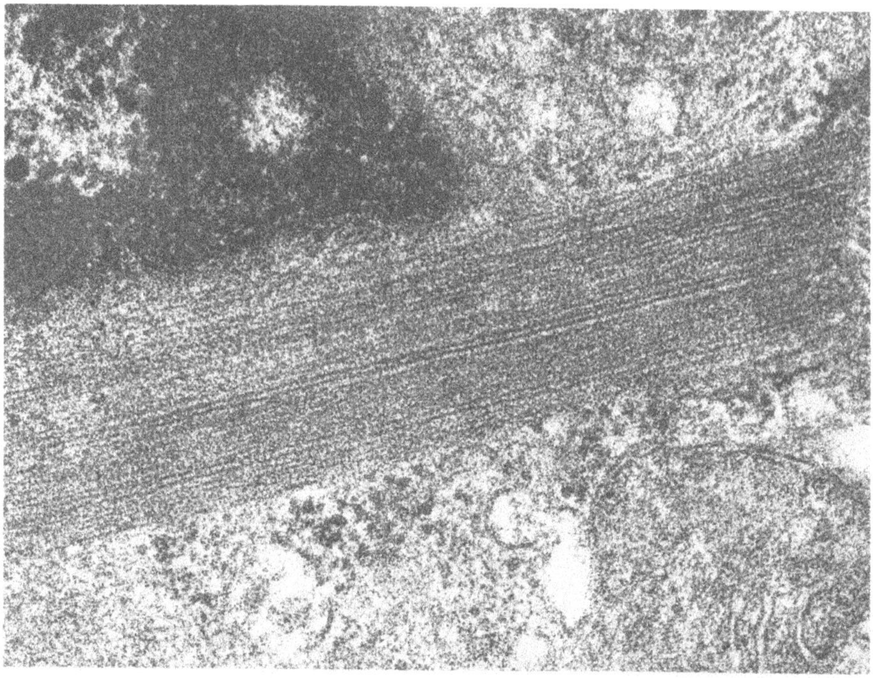

Fig. 4.22. Fibrillary inclusion. The inclusion is again seen to be composed of parallel longitudinal fibrils of 90 Å diameter, but transverse striations of similar dimensions are also seen in this plane of section. As is frequently the case, the inclusion lies in close proximity to the nucleus. The inclusions are also often closely related to the glycogen-membrane clefts illustrated in Fig. 4.15 (× 84,000)

[44]. As discussed in Sect. 5.3.2, this demonstrates that at least some latex particles are truly phagocytosed [44].

As pointed out earlier (Sect. 4.2.1), isoenzyme 5 of acid phosphatase reacts poorly with Gomori's sodium β-glycerophosphate substrate. KATAYAMA et al. [207] failed to demonstrate activity in HCs at the ultrastructural level with this substrate, but were able to find reactivity when naphthyl ASBI phosphoric acid was used as substrate. Others [5, 322], however, were able to detect TRAP activity with β-glycerophosphate as substrate, and we have found similar levels of positivity with β-glycerophosphate and naphthyl ASBI phosphoric acid as substrates.

Conventionally fixed HCs are consistently unreactive under conditions readily demonstrating myeloperoxidase activity at the ultrastructural level [93]. But it has recently been shown that, under certain reaction conditions, HCs possess an endogenous peroxidase that is distinct from myeloperoxidase [5, 311, 312]. We can confirm these observations (Fig. 4.26). This endogenous peroxidase activity is located in the perinuclear envelope and in both rough and smooth ER cisternae, but not in the Golgi apparatus or in the cytoplasmic granules. In a proportion of cases, the endogenous peroxidase activity is enhanced by short-term culture [312]. The demonstration of this activity of HCs usually requires the use of unfixed cells and high concentrations of diaminobenzidine (DAB) substrate [5]. The activity is inhibited by aminotriazole and cyanide but is not demonstrable with the alkaline DAB medium [280], which detects catalase [312]. Although its precise identity remains unknown, the endogenous peroxidase activity of HCs is clearly distinct from myeloperoxidase and catalase, and is absent

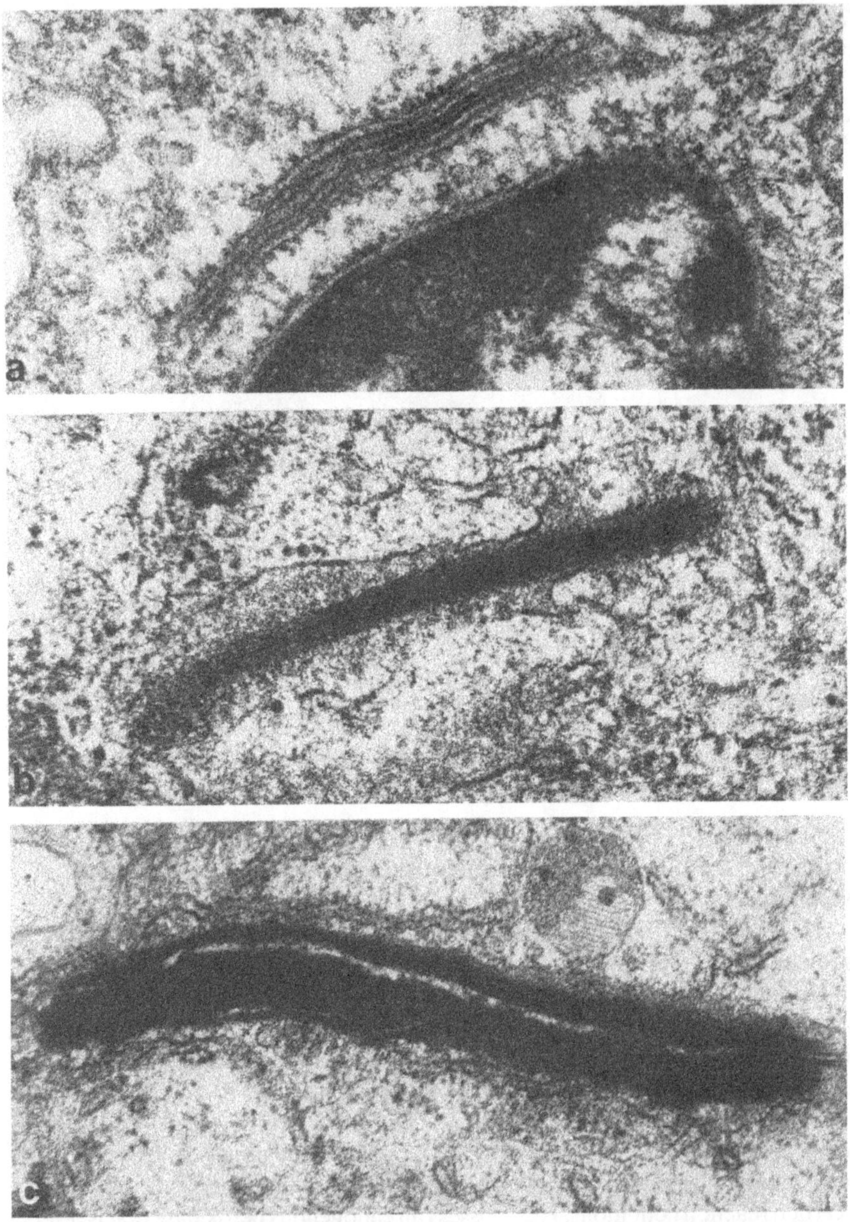

Fig. 4.23a–c. Endoplasmic reticulum (ER)-associated structures in HCs. Three apparently different types of ER-associated structure are illustrated; their nature is not clear. The mitochondrion in **c** contains a cross-hatched structure of the type reported by KATAYAMA and SCHNEIDER [203] (**a** × 55,000; **b** × 75,000; **c** × 21,000)

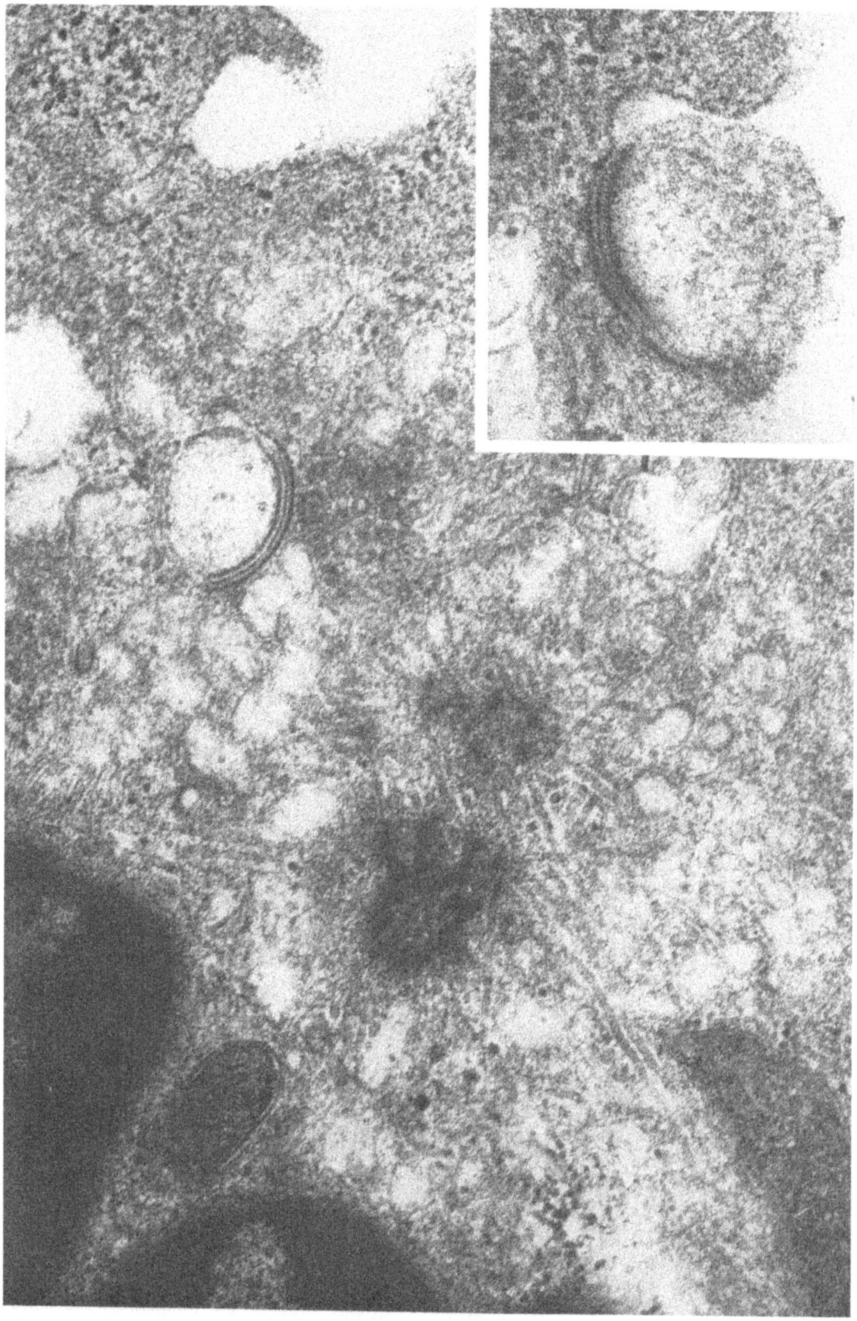

Fig. 4.24. Zipper-like junctions or Langerhans-like granules. Zipper-like junctions are seen apparently within the cell and at the cell surface (*inset*); their pentalaminar structure is shown. The centrioles, pericentriolar satellites and converging microtubules are prominent in this plane of section (× 50,000; *inset* × 78,000)

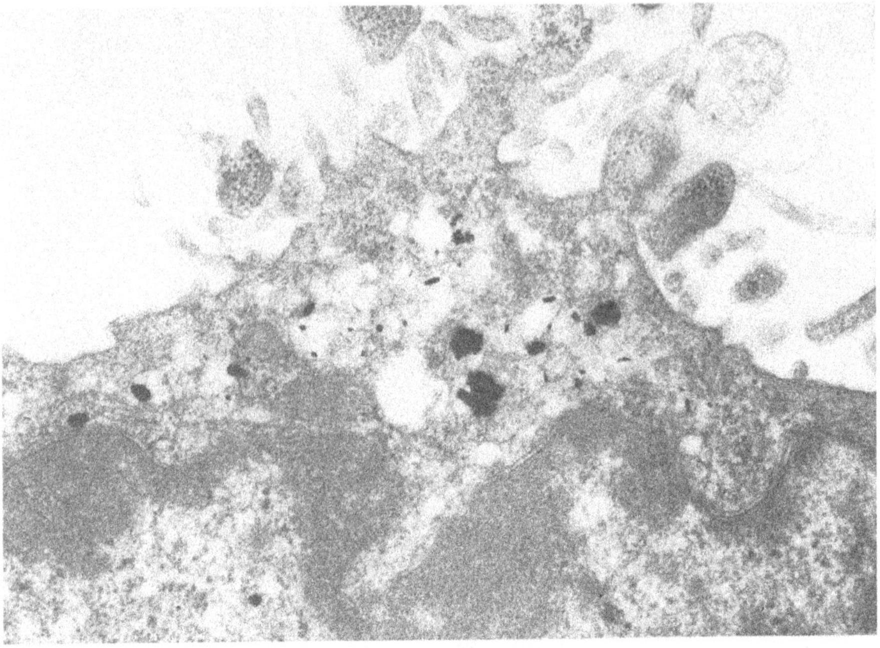

Fig. 4.25. Acid phosphatase. Enzyme activity is present in some of the granules, but a proportion of the reaction product is not clearly granule-associated (× 44,000)

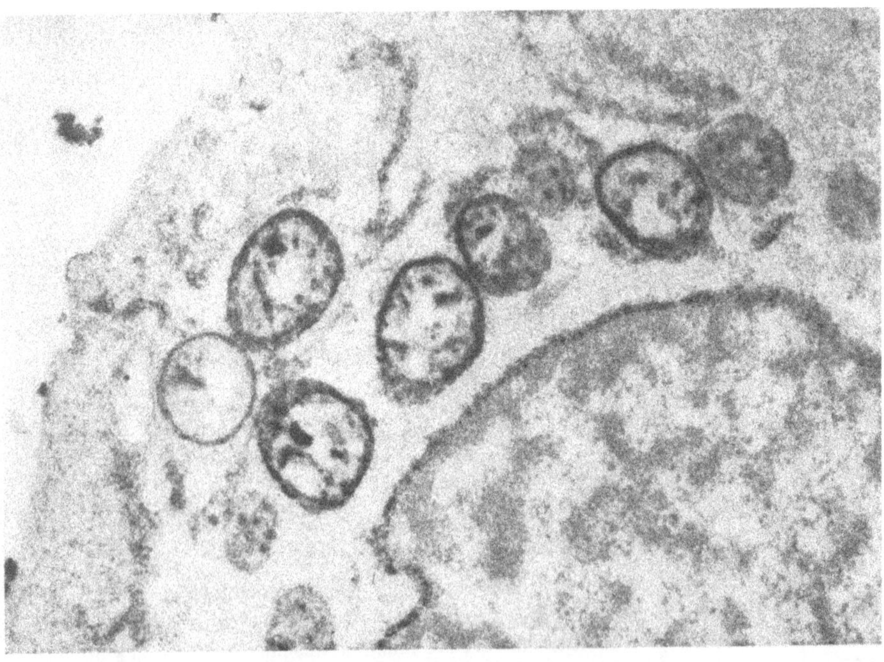

Fig. 4.26. Peroxidase. Peroxidatic activity is seen in the perinuclear cistern and in the strands of ER. The mitochondrial membranes display prominent activity attributable to cytochrome oxidase (× 36,000)

from normal and malignant B and T cells [312]. In contrast, the enzyme resembles that demonstrable in cells of the megakaryocytic series [34], in Kupffer cells and peritoneal macrophages of some animal species [92, 118], and in blood monocytes after adherence in short-term culture [25]. The significance of the endogenous peroxidase activity of HCs is, therefore, at present unclear (Sect. 5.3), but it is of interest that REYES et al. [312] found a similar peroxidatic enzyme in a small proportion of normal mononuclear cells of lymphoid appearance.

4.3.2 Scanning Electron Microscopy (SEM)

The preparative technique used has a profound effect on the surface topography of haemic cells. While many technical points are probably relevant for the optimal visualization of surface morphology (reviewed by POLLIACK [299, 301]), it is particularly important that separated cells should be rapidly fixed in suspension in an appropriate fixative, collected onto the examination surface without aspiration or filtration, and dehydrated by freeze-drying or critical-point drying methods [33, 184, 299].

As BRAYLAN et al. [33] point out, many studies of HCs are difficult to interpret, either because precise details of methodology have not been given [66, 147, 317, 336, 338] or because preparative techniques now considered suboptimal have been used [42, 148, 300, 301, 372]. Most studies, including those in which currently recommended methodology has been used [33, 94, 203], have agreed that peripheral blood HCs display prominent ruffles alone or a combination of ruffles, ridge-like projections, and narrow, finger-like microvilli (Fig. 4.27). All these different surface types can be observed with varying frequency within the same case. Although it has been claimed that splenic HCs lack ruffles and display only surface microvilli [66], our own observations and those of others [33, 102] suggest that when optimal methodology is employed there is no difference in the surface morphology of peripheral blood and splenic HCs.

A population of cells displaying a purely villous surface is usually present in mononuclear cell suspensions from both peripheral blood (Fig. 4.27d) and spleen. The identity of these cells is not entirely clear, but while some may be T cells, others are probably B cells directly involved in the clonal proliferation (Sect. 6.4.2). (For example, we have observed that a proportion of these villous cells both form SIg rosettes with a single light chain and rosette with erythrocytes coated with IgM.)

Most authors agree that the surface morphology of HCs allows no definite conclusion concerning their cell lineage, but nevertheless point out that prominent surface ruffles are a feature of normal and leukaemic monocytes, and are not observed in a range of other lymphomas or leukaemias [33, 151, 203, 286, 310].

4.4 Cytokinetics

Hairy cells are not actively dividing cells and, although they can divide, very few mitoses are seen in peripheral blood or splenic smears; the occasional mitoses in bone marrow from HCL patients can usually be identified as involving erythroid precursors. This absence of mitoses is also a constant feature of all tissues examined histologically [40]. These observations are consistent with the finding that a low percentage of HCs are in the S phase of the cell cycle [33] and with the demonstration that HCs, whether from blood, bone marrow, spleen, or liver, show little or no incorporation of tritiated thymidine [21, 33, 101, 325].

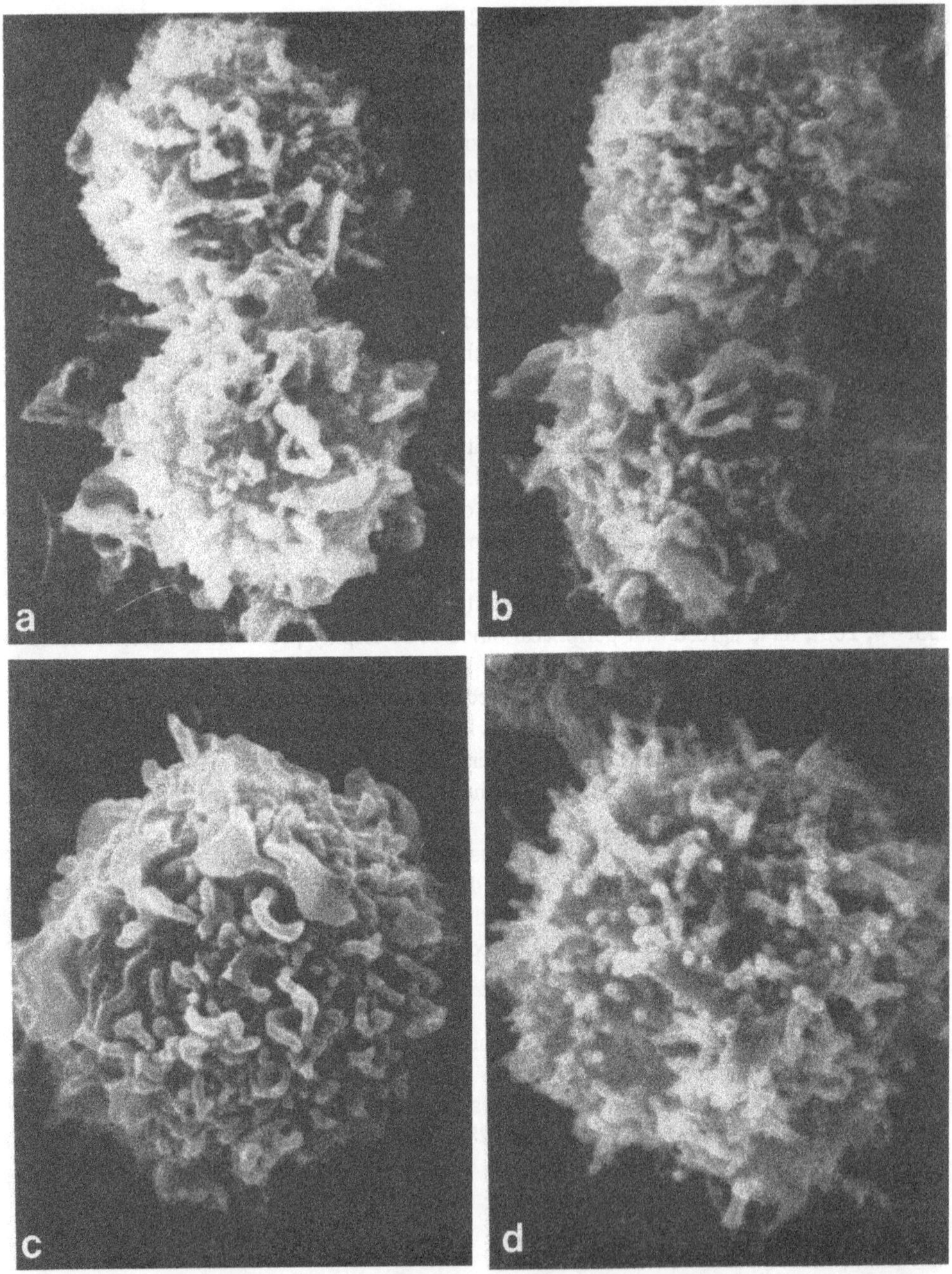

Fig. 4.27a–d. Scanning electron microscopy of HCs, illustrating the variation in the surface morphology of the peripheral blood mononuclear cells in HCL. Even within the same sample, cells displaying the hybrid feature of villi and ruffles are seen together with cells having predominantly one or other surface structure. Thus **a** shows two cells in which ruffles predominate; **b** illustrates a cell (*upper*) with mainly microvilli, together with a hybrid cell (*lower*) with ruffles and microvilli; **c** shows a hybrid cell in which microvilli are prominent, and **d** a cell exhibiting mainly microvilli (**a** × 9,500; **b** × 10,000; **c** × 12,000; **d** × 14,000)

The survival time of HCs in the circulation has not been adequately studied, although a report of a single splenectomized patient tested with tritiated cytidine has demonstrated a relatively long half-life of approximately 150 h [101]. Skin-window studies [335, 342, 385] have shown that HCs do not migrate into the skin in substantial numbers. In addition, HCs do not migrate in response to chemotactic factors in vitro [373].

4.5 Cytogenetics

The karyotype of HCs has been little studied, probably because of the few mitoses found in direct smears or in nonstimulated short-term cultures. Analysis of PHA-stimulated cultures is mostly concentrated on examination of the T lymphocytes present, and in the four cases we have studied the karyotype was normal. Unstimulated cultures of HCs do reveal a few mitoses, while the granulation, acid-phosphatase positivity and peripheral hairs show that the dividing cells are HCs (Sect. 4.7); these cells, in our experience, also show no karyotypic abnormalities even when banding is performed. KATAYAMA and FINKEL [202] found normal karyotypes in four patients examined. GOLOMB et al. [146, 150] have also found that most patients' constitutional karyotypes are normal, and these authors were able to evaluate mitoses, probably reflecting dividing HCs, in the unstimulated blood of 13 patients with HCL. Of these, two had a consistent abnormality in the majority of metaphases and five had an abnormality in a single cell. The consistent abnormality involved the absence of the Y chromosome and an added chromosome in the C group: in one case this extra chromosome was definitely identified as No. 12. It may be significant that in an earlier study of a single case, in addition to other abnormalities, two extra chromosomes were present in the C group in spreads of unstimulated splenic cells [389]. The significance of the Y-chromosome loss is difficult to assess, since loss of this chromosome is a common occurrence in normal ageing adults [282, 296].

4.6 Metabolism

Glucose utilization by HCs appears to be intermediate between that of lymphocytes and that of monocytes [43, 211], and the cells show the predominant Krebs-cycle activity [211] that might be expected from their significant mitochondrial content.

4.7 Culture

HCs can be maintained in vitro for considerable periods without necessarily constituting a cell line, and there are several reports of such cultures [9, 43, 58, 141, 286]. There is general agreement that the HCs retain their characteristic morphology and cytochemistry during a culture period of 1 or 2 months and that the cells do not mature into other cell types, particularly macrophages, during this time.

It has been suggested than on the first day of culture the cells adhere to, and spread out on, glass cover slips, with the simultaneous loss of many of the cytoplasmic hairs [286]. However, cells cultured for 2–3 weeks maintain a hairy morphology [9, 43, 58, 141], and many of these cells remain unattached in the medium. In our experience, there are glass-adherent cells in the early stages of culture but there are also many morphological HCs that remain in suspension:

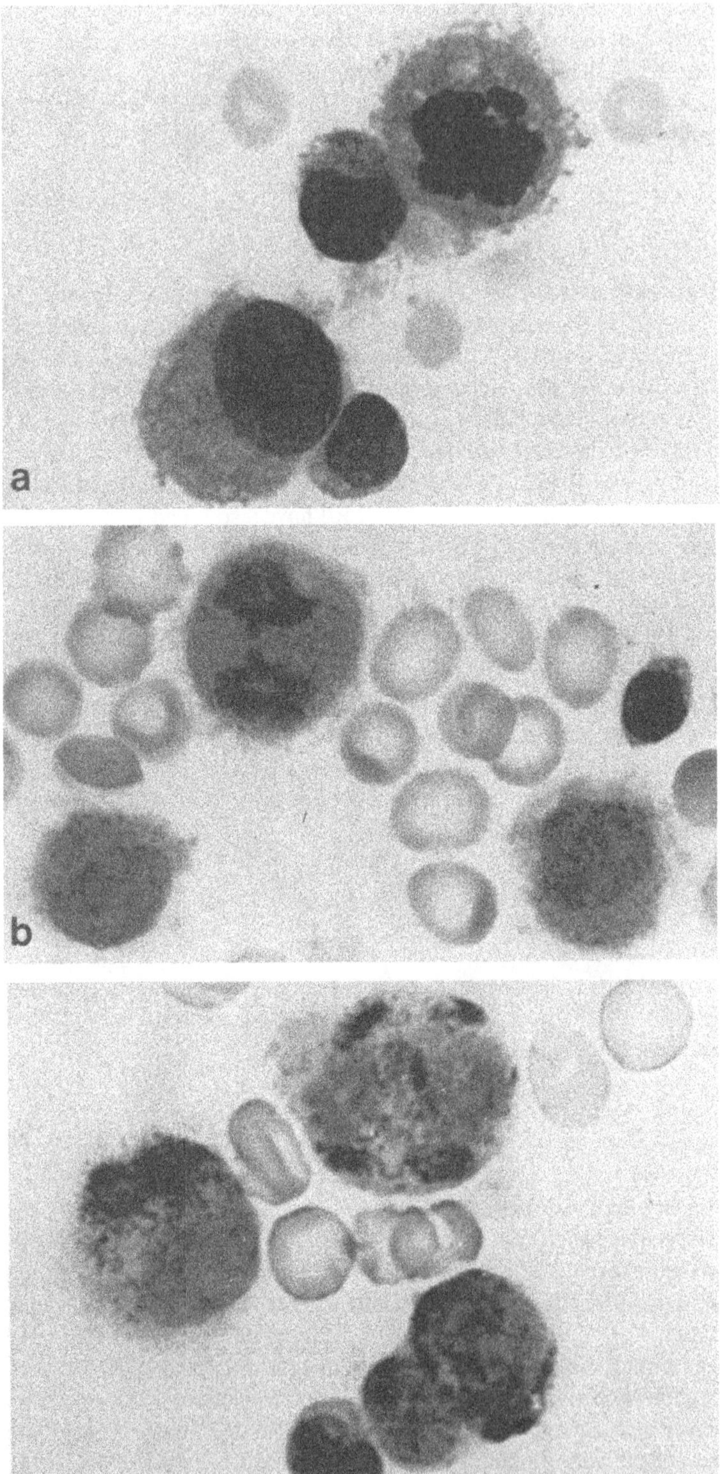

Fig. 4.28a–c

when splenic cells are cultured, some of the attached cells are fibroblasts and these may incidentally provide a feeder-layer effect for the majority HC population. The cells grow very slowly as small clusters of a few cells over the attached monolayer, and these are quite different from the large clusters typically seen in lymphoblastoid cell lines. Mitoses are uncommon but can be demonstrated in unequivocal HCs (Fig. 4.28), and the cells can also be shown to incorporate tritiated thymidine [9]. After several days of culture, HCs are seen to develop numerous cytoplasmic vacuoles [286], and the fine cytoplasmic granules present before culture become larger and markedly more abundant [286] (Fig. 4.29). It is noticeable that the granules tend to be more prominent on one side of the eccentric nucleus [286]. The cultured HCs are positive for nonspecific esterase [286], and remain strongly positive for TRAP [286] (Fig. 4.30). The cytochemical activity of the cultured cells, however, tends to be concentrated in a crescentic configuration on one side of the nucleus (Fig. 4.30). Immunologically, the cells retain the phenotype present before culture. They remain EBNA-negative [58] and retain the μFc and γFc receptors [58]; indeed, in our experience almost 100% of cultured HCs express the two Fc receptors strongly. Cultured cells from our cases did not form spontaneous rosettes with mouse erythrocytes, but strong rosette formation was observed with monkey erythrocytes (Sect. 5.2.6). The cells continue to express surface immunoglobulin of the same isotypes as before culture; thus both IgG-only cases [9, 260] and multiple heavy-chain isotype cases [58] retain their phenotype. Cytoplasmic Ig has been examined in one case (after 66 days' culture), and only a single light-chain type was detected [58]. After some time in culture

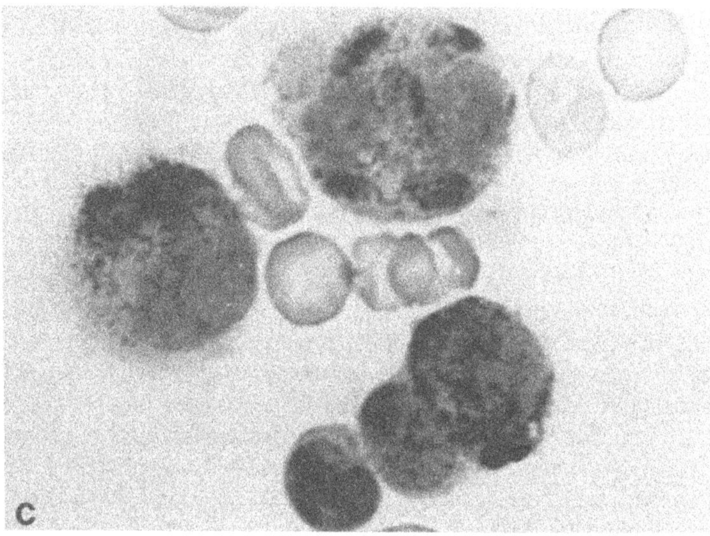

Fig. 4.29. Cultured HCs. The five HCs show increased cytoplasmic granulation. Two agranular small lymphocytes are present

---

◀ **Fig. 4.28a–c.** Mitoses in cultured HCs. **a** This ROMANOWSKY-stained preparation shows a cell with peripheral hairs in a late stage of mitosis. **b** The cell in mitosis displays the esterase staining pattern of HCs. **c** The cell in mitosis contains strong TRAP activity; the distribution of enzyme activity is characteristic of dividing HCs

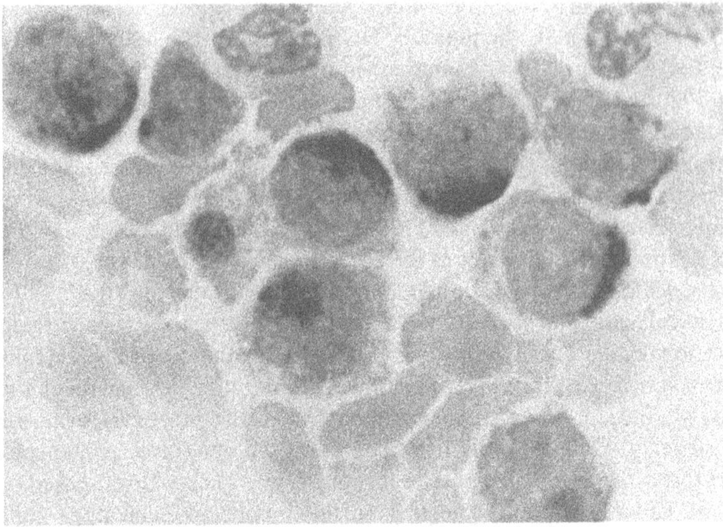

Fig. 4.30. Cultured HCs in TRAP preparation. The HCs contain strong TRAP activity, which is distributed in a crescentic configuration. Two unreactive polymorphs are present together with a probable T lymphocyte containing dot TRAP activity

the HCs show no sign of developing into macrophages [9, 58, 141, 276]. Frequently, however, numerous plasmacytoid cells are seen in the cultures [58, 286].

We and others [43] have failed to obtain established HC lines in suspension. There have been several such lines reported [144, 175, 210, 229, 260, 331, 345–347], but the details given of the cultured cells are often incomplete and contradictory, and it is therefore not possible to reach a general conclusion about the nature and significance of established HC lines.

For example, SINKOVIKS' group succeeded in establishing cell lines from the spleens of two patients with HCL [229, 345–347]. Initially, there was a natural fibroblast monolayer present but, after some 4 weeks, large clumps of lymphoid cells grew out, which did not require a feeder layer. Both cell lines were positive for TRAP, and both maintained a hairy morphology; but, remarkably, cells from both lines were seen to contain herpes-type virus particles. The cells from one of the lines were later demonstrated to be EBNA-positive, and DNA-DNA renaturation kinetic analysis demonstrated a close homology between the DNA of the virus being produced and that of the EB virus of African Burkitt's lymphoma. There was no evidence of EBV DNA in the original splenic material before culture, and the viral DNA showed less homology with American strains of EBV. The immunological phenotype of the cells changed somewhat with prolonged culture: from being SIgG-positive [345], the cultured cells lost most SIg, but some 10% became SIgM-positive [229]. The cultured cells were negative for EAC rosettes, but were positive in the Raji test for complement receptors [229].

From 174 attempts, von HEYDEN et al. [175] were successful in establishing eight cell lines from the peripheral blood of two patients with HCL. The cells were not tested for EBNA, but after 6 weeks in culture they became negative for TRAP.

A cell line has also been established from the peripheral blood of a curious case of HCL [210]. This patient had numerous plasma cells in her peripheral blood, which were demonstrated to contain type A oncornavirus-like particles [289]. Upon culture, the peripheral blood cells grew as a monolayer of fibroblastoid cells interspersed with cells of a plasmacytoid morphology. Free-floating lymphocytoid cells produced during the early stages of culture degenerated and died off.

GOLDE's group [144, 331] have established lymphoblastoid cell lines from the peripheral blood of two cases of HCL and from the spleen of a patient with the T-cell variant of the disease. Both the B-cell lines grew rapidly as typical lymphoblastoid cell clumps after only 30 days of culture, and feeder-cell monolayers were not required. One of the B-cell lines was established from a patient with macroglobulinaemia and the cells, which had a number of atypical features (Sect. 5.4.3), maintained the same phenotype during culture. The T-cell line also maintained its orginal phenotype, but the other B-lymphoblastoid cell line, while remaining positive for TRAP, underwent a transformation in the immunoglobulin phenotype expressed and secreted by the cells (from IgGλ to IgMκ).

Since almost all B-lymphoblastoid cell lines are the result of EB virus infection and the outgrowth of permissive B lymphocytes, whatever original cell type is being cultured [198], it seems likely that many of the established lines grown from HCL specimens are in fact of this kind. Such an explanation would account for many of the apparent discrepancies in morphology and cytochemistry noted above, and also for the phenotypic changes observed with time. Furthermore, the presence of TRAP in cultured cells is not proof of an HC lineage, since we have observed TRAP in some typical B-lymphoblastoid cell lines not derived from HCL and since transformed T cells may also contain this isoenzyme [235].

5 The Hairy Cell: Immunological Aspects

5.1 Transformation and Cytotoxicity Studies

5.1.1 Mitogen-Induced Transformation

The interpretation of this type of study of peripheral blood is particularly difficult in HCL since HCs are present in variable, but frequently low, numbers, while mitogen-responsive T lymphocytes often predominate: the transformation of T cells in the disease is considered in Sect. 6.4.1 and the present section considers only the response of HCs. Two approaches have been used in attempts to overcome the problem of T-cell contamination. In the first, "pure" HC populations have been obtained from the peripheral blood of floridly leukaemic cases [27, 69] or from spleen [96, 211, 389], or by employing glass-adherent cells [101]. In the second approach, attempts have been made to identify the origin of the transformed cells by a number of methods: by E-rosette formation [166]; by TRAP staining [314]; or, in this laboratory, by the presence of R-L complexes at the ultrastructural level.

Most such studies have led to the conclusion that the majority of HCs show little or no transformation in response to any mitogens [69, 96, 101, 164, 166, 211, 322, 328, 375, 389], including specific antigens [211], but that pokeweed mitogen (PWM) may be a slightly better stimulator than phytohaemagglutinin (PHA) [314]. Occasional HCs can be shown to have undergone transformation in response to PHA [69, 213], PWM and Lima-bean lectin [314]. Such transformed HCs have been positively identified by TRAP reactivity [314] and, in our own studies, by the observation of R-L complexes in occasional blast cells (Fig. 5.1).

There are reports in which unfractionated peripheral blood mononuclear cells from some cases of HCL respond in a biphasic manner to PHA [27, 272, 325] or PWM [69]. The biphasic response, which is similar to that observed in peripheral blood cultures from CLL [65, 69, 324], consists of a minimal blastic transformation on day 3 followed by a peak response on days 5–7. This delayed response has been interpreted in different ways: some authors [27] suggest that it represents a proliferation of HCs, while others [272] consider it to be a late response by the normal T cells present. By pulse-chase labelling, Rubin et al. [325] demonstrated that in HCL an appreciable number of the blasts observed in the second peak were the result of a replication and enlargement of the PHA-responsive lymphocyte population seen in the earlier peak.

5.1.2 Mixed Lymphocyte Reactions (MLR)

HCs have the capacity to serve as stimulator cells in one-way allogeneic MLR [27, 96, 213, 272]. In some cases the stimulating capacity of both peripheral blood [272] and splenic [96] HCs in MLR is much poorer than that of control cells. The reason for their poor stimulating capacity is unknown, but CLL cells are also poor stimulators in MLR [349], despite the fact that both HCs and CLL cells express readily detectable Ia-like antigen on the cell surface (Sect. 5.2.6). Since the Ia antigen is the stimulating component in MLR, it is of interest that

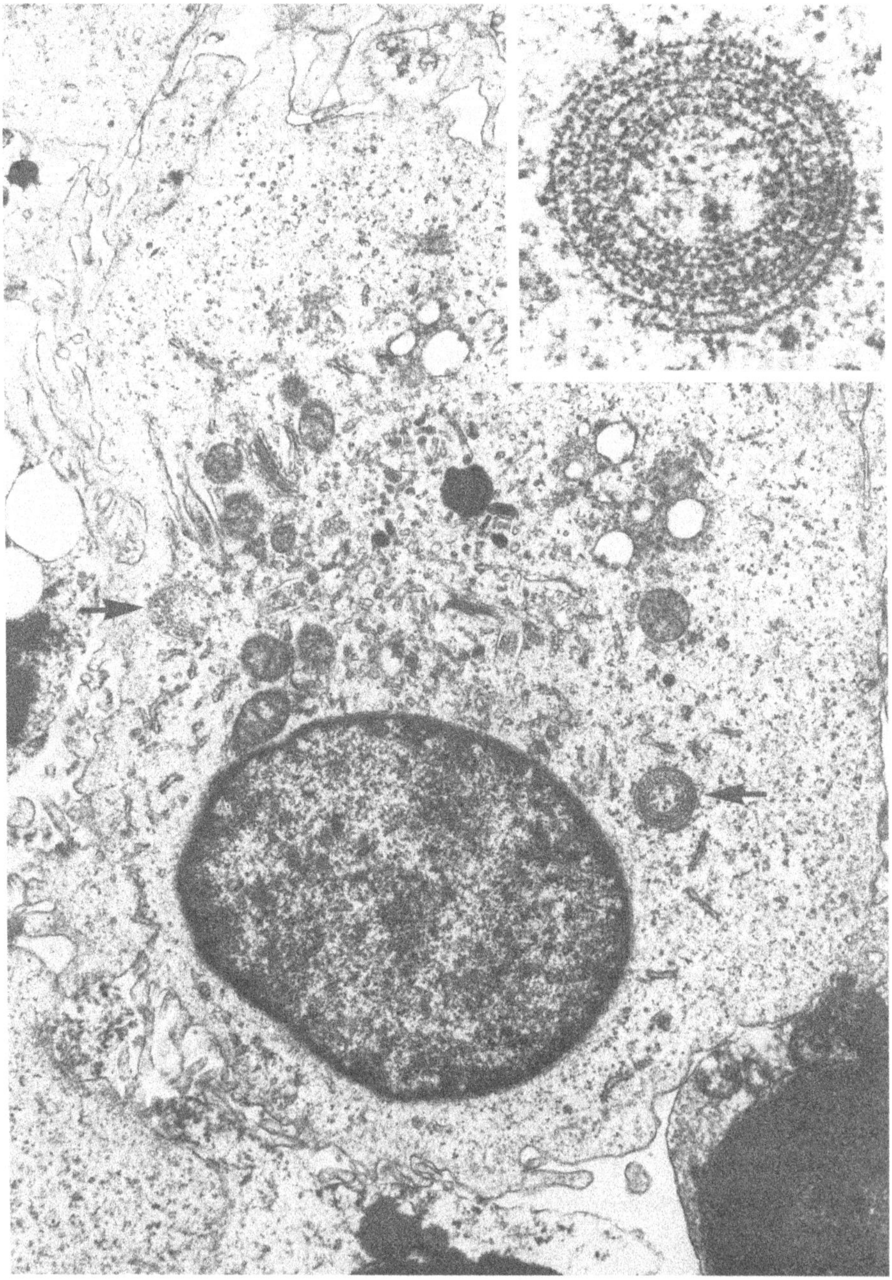

Fig. 5.1. Transformed HC. This PHA-transformed blast cell contains two R-L complexes (↑) and is presumably therefore derived from a hairy cell (× 13,000). The transversely sectioned complex is shown at higher power in the *inset* and its typical fine structure is demonstrated (× 61,000)

HCs from a case of T-cell HCL, which did not express the Ia-like antigen, also served as stimulator cells in the MLR [272].

When allowance is made for contaminating T lymphocytes, HCs show little or no transformation response to allogeneic lymphocytes [27, 96, 213].

Non-T lymphocytes from normal human peripheral blood can stimulate autologous T cells to proliferate in a one-way MLR [222]. Splenic HCs did not stimulate autologous splenic T cells in this reaction, even though the T cells functioned normally in an allogeneic MLR [96].

5.1.3 Cytotoxicity Functions

The ability of HCs to act as effector cells in various cytotoxic assay systems has been little studied, but they appear to be unable to effect allogeneic cell-mediated lympholysis (a T-cell function [27]). Their activity against IgG-coated erythrocytes in the antibody-dependent cell-mediated cytotoxicity test (a K-cell function) is weak [328] or absent [3, 27, 63]. In the lectin-induced cellular cytotoxicity test (a function of most mononuclear cells including monocytes), HCs can function as cytotoxic effector cells when pretreated with either PHA [328] or wheat germ agglutinin [27].

5.2 Surface Receptors

5.2.1 Sheep Erythrocyte (E) Rosettes and Anti-T Cell Sera

In general, HCs do not form spontaneous rosettes with sheep erythrocytes (E rosettes). As in normal blood, therefore, E-rosette formation in HCL is a reliable indicator of circulating T-cell proportions. The use of sheep erythrocytes that have been pretreated with neuraminidase or aminoethylisothiouronium bromide [197] avoids the problem of the weakly avid T cells occasionally found in chronic leukaemias [277, 380]. In our experience, the peripheral blood and splenic HCs of three entirely typical cases of HCL did not stain with a rabbit anti-T cell serum (raised against monkey thymocytes [160]), which stains most normal human peripheral T cells. The percentage of mononuclear cells staining with this serum closely correlated with that forming E rosettes [77]; but, in many cases of HCL, we have observed occasional unequivocal HCs forming E rosettes. This observation may simply reflect the inherent stickiness of HCs [44], but it may be of more general significance, since several cases of HCL have now been described in which a high proportion of HCs formed E rosettes and reacted with an anti-T cell serum (Sect. 5.6). Moreover, STEIN and KAISERLING [361] have observed that the HCs of their two cases stained with a specific anti-thymocyte serum.

5.2.2 Surface Immunoglobulin (SIg)

The evidence that HCs express genuine intrinsic SIg of restricted light-chain type is now compelling. The monoclonal SIg comprises either IgG alone [2, 33, 58, 63, 88, 131, 191, 213, 227, 315, 316, 352] or multiple heavy-chain isotypes [27, 33, 58, 77, 102, 129, 164, 166, 191, 213, 315, 316, 361].

Until recently, SIg expression by HCs has been a controversial issue, for a number of reasons. For example, the strong γFc receptor on HCs (see below) has often been invoked to account for the varied, and frequently multiple, heavy-chain isotypes of SIg reported on HCs [63, 185, 211, 341]. Indeed, work showing polyclonal (κ and λ) SIg patterns [13, 158, 211, 304, 310, 361, 395] is probably explicable in terms of Fc binding. Also, because of the unusual nature of the SIg on HCs, proof of its intrinsic nature has required special attention to the various technical aspects of SIg detection. Thus, particularly for SIgG, the possibility must be excluded that apparent SIg might be caused by labile extrinsic autologous IgG (whether autoantibody or immunoglobulin bound to γFc receptors [179, 382]) or by heterologous reagent binding. In addition, the specificity of the reagents used for SIg detection is crucially important. We have examined the complete SIg phenotype of peripheral blood HCs from 26 cases of HCL. Some of the cases were studied by direct immunofluorescence with affinity-purified antisera, and all cases were examined by a direct agglutination rosette method (Fig. 5.2). In this method, which is more sensitive than direct immunofluorescence [165], purified sheep IgG against individual human heavy and light chains is coupled by chromic chloride to indicator ox erythrocytes [58, 237]. Restricted light-chain expression (18κ, 8λ) was seen in all the cases, and this indicates the probable monoclonality of HCL. With regard to heavy-chain isotype expression, the cases fell into two main groups. In half the patients (13 cases) the cells expressed only IgG (10κ, 3λ). The cells in all the other cases displayed two, three, or four heavy-chain isotypes, but invariably showed restricted light chain expression. All 13 multiple isotype cases expressed SIgD as the predominant or copredominant heavy-chain isotype, and the percentage of $SIgD^+$ cells closely approximated to that of cells bearing the exclusive light-chain type. The expression of other heavy-chain isotypes (MGA) was variable, but SIgM was frequently expressed on a relatively small percentage of cells (parallel tests with CLL cells demonstrated that this low level of IgM expression was not due to technical factors). In all these mixed cases, the sum of two or more heavy-chain isotypes greatly exceeded both the percentage of cells bearing the exclusive light-chain type and the percentage of Fc^+E^- (non-T) cells. This indicates that two or more heavy-chain isotypes were simultaneously expressed on

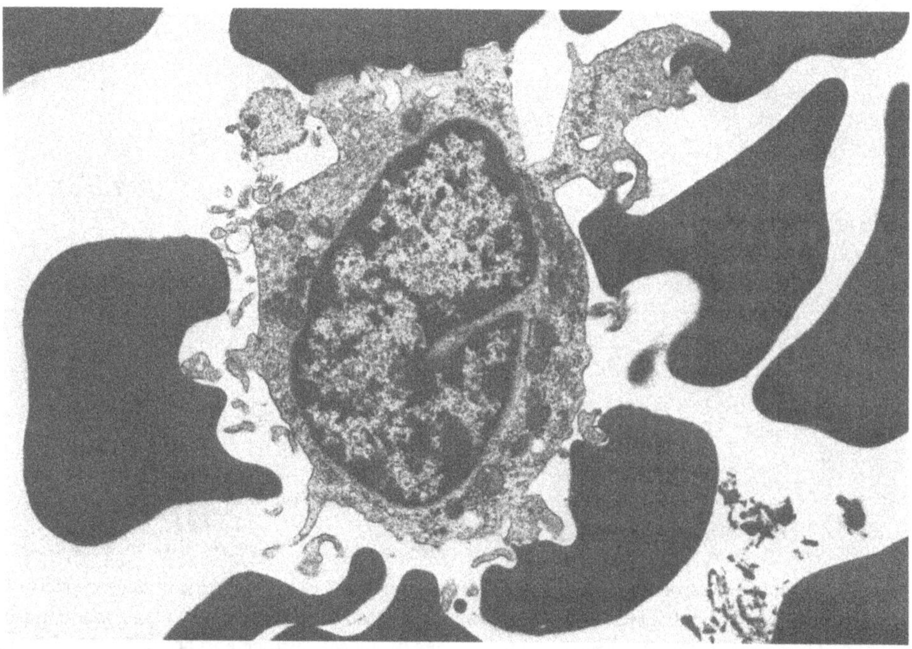

Fig 5.2. Transmission electron microscopy of SIgD rosette. The HC is clearly rosetting with the ox erythrocytes coupled to sheep anti-human IgD (× 8,000)

the same cell. The detailed heavy-chain phenotypes of our multiple isotype cases are given in Table 5.1. Recently, broadly similar results have been obtained by JANSEN et al. [191], who employed fluorescent staining of formaldehyde-fixed HCs, and by RIEBER et al. [315, 316] with autoradiography.

We have also examined the SIg phenotype of the splenic HCs from 11 of our cases and, in all but one, it was identical with that of the peripheral blood HCs. In the one exception, the splenic HCs expressed only SIgD, while those in the peripheral blood were $D^+G^+A^+$. We have also examined bone-marrow HCs from five cases, and the phenotype was again identical with that

Table 5.1. Detailed SIg phenotype of HCs in patients[a] showing multiple heavy-chain isotype expression

Heavy-chain isotypes	DM (1)	DG (1)	DGM (7)	DGA (1)	DGMA (3)
Light-chain isotypes	κ	κ	κ (2) λ (5)	κ	κ (3)
Relative preponderance of individual heavy-chain isotypes	D = M	D > G	D = G = M (1) D = G > M (2) D > G > M (4)	D > G > A	D = A > M > G (1) D > A > M > G (2)

[a] The figures in parentheses give the numbers of cases

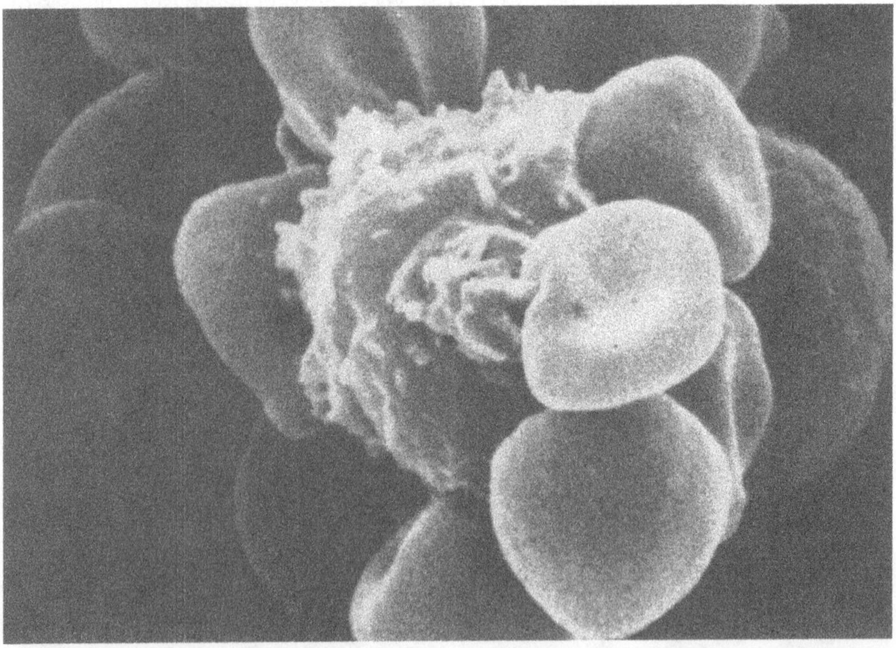

Fig. 5.3. Scanning electron microscopy of SIgG rosette. Many of the rosetting indicator cells are localized towards one pole of the HC, and at least one can be seen to be associated with a pseudopod-like extension. The red cells are attached over broad areas of the cell surface and are distinctly deformed at points of attachment. As is often the case, the opposite pole of the HC appears relatively denuded of both microvilli and ruffles (× 10,500)

of peripheral blood cells. In contrast, in the only case in which we have been able to examine lymph-node material, the γFc^+E^- HCs were largely SIg-negative, although the few SIg^+ cells were of the same phenotype (Gκ) as the peripheral blood, bone-marrow and spleen cells. However, SIg negativity is not confined to lymph-node HCs and a few examples of SIg-negative cases have been reported [191, 333]. We have not observed consistently negative cases, but have noted wide fluctuations in SIg expression by the HCs of some patients.

When HCs are stained for SIg by immunofluorescent methods, we and others [33, 102, 129, 314, 327, 328] have frequently observed that the SIg appears to be localized at one pole. This is presumably due to rapid capping and occurs even when the test is carried out at 4° C in the presence of azide. This rapid capping is a particular feature of HCs and is not seen in other cell types. The same phenomenon is observed at the ultrastructural level when SIg is detected by immunoperoxidase staining [327, 328] or by rosette formation; this is shown in Figs. 5.3 and 5.4, where most of the rosetting erythrocytes can be seen to be localized to one pole of the cell, with the cytoplasm forming a pseudopod-like extension.

Because of the importance of technical considerations in the study of SIg, this aspect of our investigations requires emphasis. A routine preincubation step at 37° C was employed to remove autoantibody. Detection of extrinsic autologous γFc-bound IgG is unlikely to show the restricted light-chain pattern consistently observed in our study. Furthermore, SIg persisted unaltered in the 12 cases tested after short-term culture (12 h to 4 days) and after more prolonged periods in vitro (Sect. 4.7: Culture). The problem of heterologous reagent binding to the γFc receptor was overcome by the use of the rosette method for SIg detection [58, 165]. Furthermore, we have demonstrated the intrinsic nature of the SIg on HCs by showing re-expression of the different individual heavy-chain isotypes after capping and

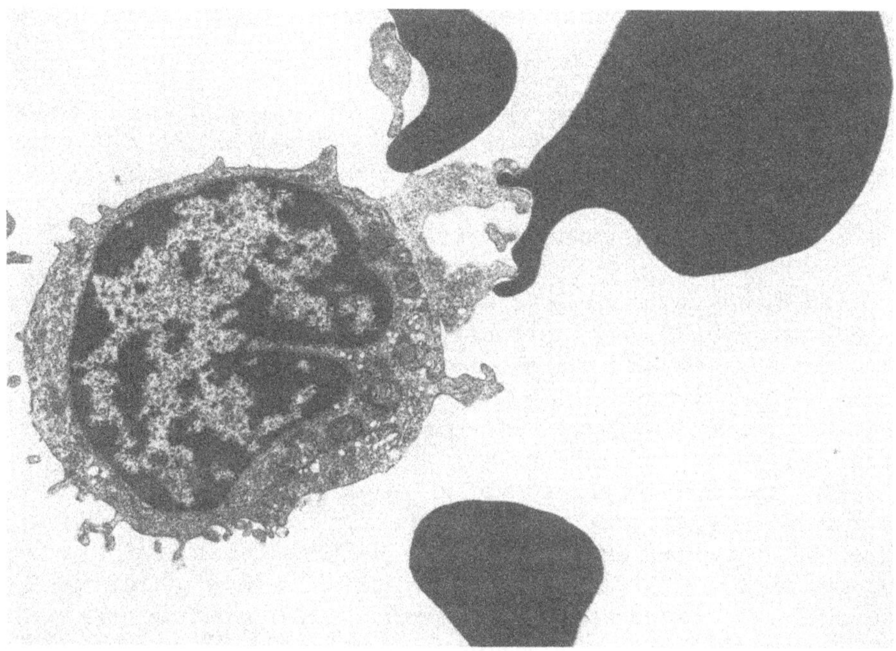

Fig. 5.4. Transmission electron microscopy of SIgD rosette. The prominent pseudopod-like extensions at one pole of the HC are firmly attached to deformed indicator erythrocytes (× 10,000)

stripping with anti-Ig reagents [58, 80]. The time taken for re-expression was in excess of 18 h [58, 80], and this is in agreement with other studies in which the same method of Ig stripping was employed [314, 316]. There have been reports of shorter re-expression times after removal of SIg by trypinization [213, 227, 375]; but the SIg may not have been completely removed, since we and others [33, 316] have been unable to remove SIg completely with trypsin or papain without killing the HCs. The specificity of the antisera used in our study was extensively tested by microagglutination of erythrocytes coupled to purified myeloma proteins and by indirect immunofluorescence on a complete panel of different myeloma cell types. In addition, the use of the same antisera for a large number of patients provided an internal control for cross-reactivity.

Our SIg findings in HCL can be contrasted with those in CLL. Thus investigators employing both the sensitive rosette method and direct immunofluorescence [58, 90, 105, 165, 193, 304], have shown the following points of difference: the majority of CLL cases express SIgM and SIgD only; the level of SIgM expression is much higher in CLL (approximating to that of SIgD); SIgG-only cases of CLL are uncommon; SIg-negative cases of CLL are frequent; SIgA is very rare.

5.2.3 Fc Receptors

HCs have receptors for the Fc of IgE (εFc), the Fc of IgG (γFc), and the Fc of IgM (μFc).

εFc. In a single report [352], one of two cases of HCL was positive for an εFc receptor. The possible significance of this receptor is unknown, but εFc receptors have been reported to occur on subpopulations of normal B and T cells [152, 392] and have also been observed on lymphosarcoma cells, but not on the cells of Sézary's syndrome or acute lymphoblastic leukaemia (ALL) [352].

γFc. Most studies of HCL agree that HCs have receptors for γFc [33, 49, 63, 129, 166, 185, 191, 375]. The methods used to detect the receptor have varied, and some reports have concluded that the strong γFc receptor on HCs is evidence that these cells belong to the monocyte-histiocyte series [185, 211]. A full consideration of the nature of the γFc receptor of HCs will be given below in an examination of the monocytic features of HCL.

μFc. A large proportion of the HCs from all but one of our 25 patients tested have been shown to possess a receptor for μFc. The receptor can be found on cells from the peripheral blood, bone marrow, spleen, and lymph nodes, and on cultured HCs. Unlike the μFc receptor present on certain normal [251, 263] and pathological [264, 384] T cells, the receptor is expressed on cells without culture in serum-enriched medium, and cells bearing the receptor simultaneously express the γFc receptor.

The μFc receptor is readily demonstrated with a rosette system employing ox erythrocytes coated with a subagglutinating level of rabbit anti-ox erythrocyte IgM obtained by sephadex chromatography. Details of the reagents used and the method employed have been documented [47, 49, 51]. Blocking of the receptor is better achieved with IgM that has been monomerized or stapled by reaction with its specific antigen than with whole pentameric IgM [47, 51], and the $Fc_5\mu$ fragment of the Fc region is involved in the binding reaction [47, 122]. Aggregated IgM does not block the rosette reaction, probably because in this form the $Fc_5\mu$ region is not exposed for binding.

The characteristic morphology of the μFc rosettes formed by HCs is illustrated in Fig. 5.5. The point attachments seen in this type of rosette appear to be mainly at the ends of the fine cytoplasmic hairs and may be the result of low receptor density on the HC surface; certainly, the rosettes are very easily disrupted by rough handling during processing. Morphological examination also confirmed that very few cells other than HCs form μFc rosettes. The few

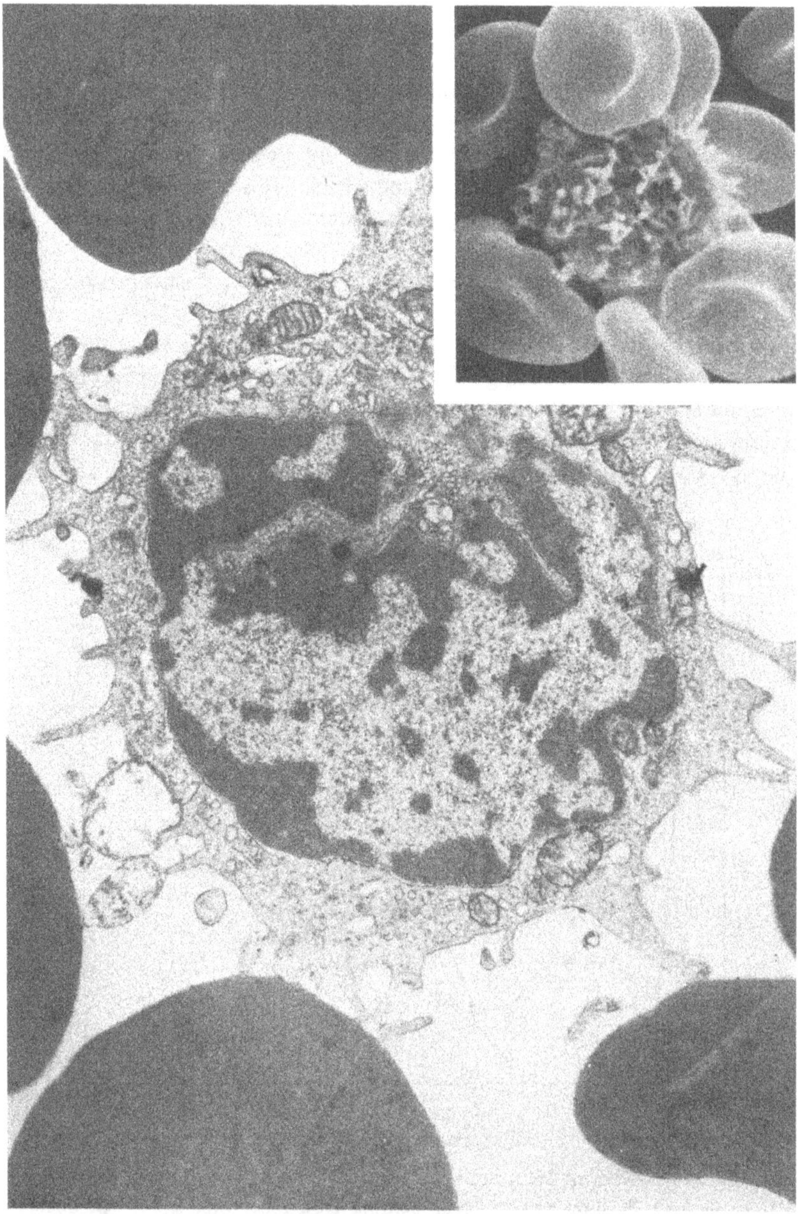

Fig. 5.5. Transmission electron microscopy of HC forming μFc rosette (× 15,000); *inset* SEM of villous HC forming μFc rosette (× 5,000). The rosetting indicator cells make point contact mainly with surface microvilli, and are not markedly deformed

monocytes and polymorphonuclear leucocytes present in rosetted preparations were invariably negative. Occasional platelets were seen to form μFc rosettes, however.

We have frequently observed that only a proportion of the HCs in a given case form μFc rosettes. This lack of receptor expression can often be attributed to receptor loss during in vitro handling of the cells, and with due attention to technical precautions nearly all peripheral blood HCs can usually be shown to possess the receptor. However, genuine fluctuations in μFc receptor expression by peripheral blood HCs do occur, since on some occasions of testing, particularly in the immediate post-splenectomy period (Fig. 5.6), many of the HCs failed to form rosettes.

Even with careful technique, a consistently lower percentage (50%) of splenic HCs formed μFc rosettes in 14 cases. These splenic cells are nevertheless capable of expressing the μFc receptor, since virtually 100% of splenic HCs are positive after short-term culture. In our only case in which both peripheral blood and splenic HCs completely lacked the receptor before culture, the majority of splenic HCs became μFc receptor-positive after 2 days' culture.

If freshly isolated HCs are washed and held either at room temperature or at 37° C in medium that does not contain serum, they rapidly lose their ability to form μFc rosettes [47]. The supernatant from such cultures will block rosette formation by other HCs, and this has been interpreted as receptor shedding [47, 49]. The presence of serum in the culture medium prevents receptor shedding [47]. The rapid shedding of μFc receptor in the absence of serum probably accounts for a reported failure to detect the receptor on HCs without culture [122]. HCs maintained in serum-free medium progressively regenerate the μFc receptor after about 6 h,

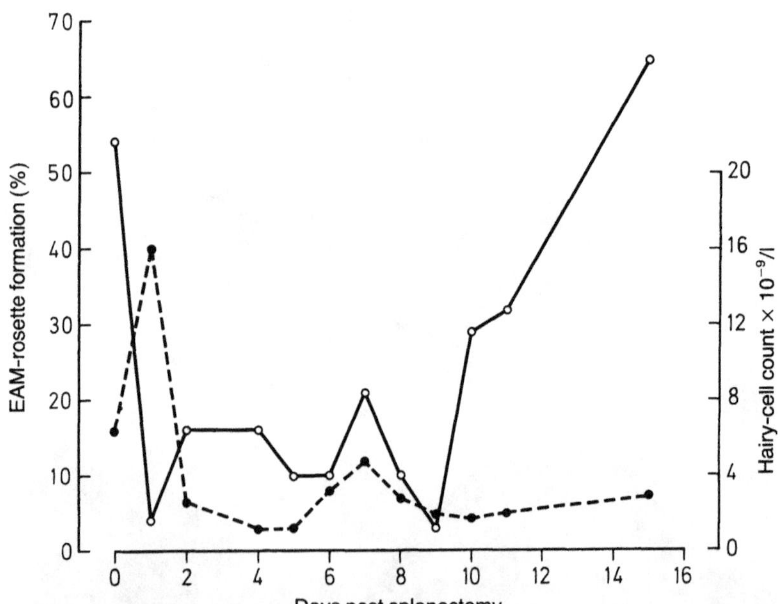

Fig. 5.6. Morphological HCs and μFc-receptor bearing cells in the immediate post-splenectomy period. ○—○, % mononuclear cells bearing μFc receptors; ●----●, absolute count of morphological HCs. In the immediate post-splenectomy period, HCs are transiently increased in number but lack μFc receptors. Later, when circulating HC numbers become stabilized, most possess μFc receptors

and this process of shedding and regeneration is repeated cyclically with a peak-to-peak re-expression time of some 6 h [49]. The regeneration process can be prevented by inhibitors of protein synthesis, and the time taken for each cycle probably reflects the membrane turnover time of HCs [49]. By the same method, the membrane turnover time of CLL cells (12 h or greater) is more than double that of HCs [49, 56].

The μFc receptor detectable without culture is absent from the cells of most human leukaemias, lymphomas and allied disorders [52] and, apart from HCL, only CLL has a significant proportion of cells that express the receptor [14, 52, 72, 122, 293, 294, 318]. Only a small percentage of normal B lymphocytes express the μFc receptor without culture, although most seem to express the receptor after culture [122, 292]. It is not yet clear, therefore, whether the possession of this receptor relates HCL and CLL to particular subpopulation(s) of normal B cells.

The function of the μFc receptor of B cells is unknown, but it does not play any role in phagocytosis [51]. It is likely, however, that the receptor has some immunological significance, since a similar μFc receptor on T cells characterizes a morphologically [24, 161] and functionally [266] distinct subpopulation of T cells. Whatever its function, the μFc receptor is of diagnostic value in distinguishing HCL from non-Hodgkin's lymphomata.

5.2.4 Receptors for Fixed C3 and the Epstein-Barr Virus

C3 Receptors. The cells from most cases of HCL do not have receptors for the third component of complement, fixed C3.

There have been conflicting reports concerning the presence of this receptor on HCs [63], but technical difficulties may have accounted for some of the work claiming to show that HCs do possess a C3 receptor [50]. Thus, most reports [63, 69, 166] have used a test system involving rosette formation with ox erythrocytes coated with IgM and complement (EAMC). With this system, the IgM receptor of HCs (μFc receptor) is able to bind the test reagent, and the complement coat serves only to reduce subsequent rosette formation. We have consistently found that the control system for complement binding – ox erythrocytes coated with IgM alone – gives a higher score than is obtained when complement is present, whether as C3b or C3d [50]. Moreover, purified monomerized IgM will block apparent complement rosette formation [50].

Further proof that apparent rosette formation with EAMC is caused by μFc-receptor binding is obtained by electron microscopy. In our studies of apparent complement rosettes formed between HCs and EAMC, the morphology of the rosettes closely resembled that illustrated by Catovsky [63]. The morphology of these rosettes closely resembled that of μFc rosettes and differed markedly from the EAC rosettes formed by normal B lymphocytes, in which the rosetting indicator cells make contact with extensive areas of the lymphocyte surface [20].

Because of the μFc receptor, tests for the detection of C3 receptors on HCs must avoid conditions allowing IgM binding. We have employed yeast particles coated directly with C3b by alternative pathway complement activation and have found that the cells from all but one of 11 cases of HCL were negative [50]. Others [63] have utilized human erythrocytes coated directly with C3b (prepared in low-ionic-strength serum to avoid the presence of IgM) to show that nine cases of HCL lacked a C3b receptor. Sheep erythrocytes probably do not bind sufficient IgM for μFc-receptor binding to occur [50], and there are several reports that sheep erythrocytes coated with IgM and complement do not form rosettes with HCs [33, 102, 151, 185, 191, 211, 249, 343]. Similarly, monolayers of glass-adherent HCs do not bind C3-coated particles under conditions permitting monocytes to do so [44, 395]. Cryostat sections of HCL spleens fail to bind C3-coated erythrocytes, although the B-lymphocyte areas of spleens from patients with nodular lymphomas firmly bind similar reagents [44, 185, 191, 249, 343, 363]. HCs do not bind IgM-coated ox erythrocytes in either monolayers or cryostat sections [44].

Thus the evidence is overwhelming that most cases of HCL lack receptors for complement. Nevertheless, there are occasional reports of HCL cases with C3 receptor-bearing HCs in which the results cannot be attributed to technical factors [27, 33, 143, 333], although some of these cases are unusual in a number of respects [27, 143]. One of our patients had HCs that formed rosettes with complement-coated erythrocytes. The patient was clinically and haematologically typical, but the HCs lacked receptors for μFc. Whether there is a direct link between μFc and C3 receptor expression awaits further study, but it may be significant that in CLL, the only other haemic malignancy in which a large number of the cells express a μFc receptor [52], the cells lack a receptor for C3b [321].

A variety of explanations have been proposed to explain the absence of C3 receptors on HCs. SHEVACH's group [185, 343] have shown that splenic macrophages, in contrast to macrophages from other sites, do not express receptors for C3, and they suggest that HCs derive from the same cell type as splenic macrophages. JANSEN et al. [191] draw attention to murine studies indicating that the environment of the spleen is necessary for B cells to acquire the C3 receptor [326], and suggest that HCs are not properly handled by the grossly deranged spleen of HCL. Perhaps a simpler theory is that HCs, regardless of cell lineage, represent a stage of development at which C3 receptors are not expressed.

Epstein-Barr Virus Receptors. HCs have not been directly studied for the presence of a receptor for the Epstein-Barr virus (EBV), but indirect evidence suggests that they lack this receptor.

The lack of receptors for complement on HCs also suggests that these cells lack EBV receptors, since there is a close relationship between C3 receptors and this virus receptor on human B cells [194, 391]. Further indirect evidence for the lack of EBV receptors on HCs comes from cell culture studies. The ability to "immortalize" cells is a feature of EBV infection, and Epstein-Barr nuclear antigen (EBNA)-negative haematological cell lines are difficult to establish [196]. Hairy-cell lines have also proved difficult to establish (see Sect. 4.7). Our only long-term primary culture of HCs remained EBNA-negative [58], but there is a single report of EBNA-positive cultures retaining HC morphology [229]. These observations suggest that the majority of HCs do not permit EBV infection with subsequent immortalization.

Attempts were made to infect our HC culture with EBV. Following the addition of virus, an outgrowth of a different cell type occurred after more than 2 weeks' culture. These EBV-infected cells grew rapidly in large clusters and rapidly replaced the morphologically typical HCs. The resulting culture was a typical lymphoblastoid cell line, and the cells differed markedly from the original cultured HCs, both morphologically and immunologically. Thus, most of the lymphoblastoid cells expressed a receptor for C3b, but were negative for the γFc and μFc receptors, and did not express SIg. Although the possibility cannot be excluded that the HCs were infected and totally transformed by EBV, the time taken for the EBV-infected line to grow out, as well as the major morphological and marker differences from HCs, suggest that this line was an outgrowth of a minority population of EBV-permissive B cells. Most haematological cell lines are of this type and are EBNA- and C3-positive, no matter what the initial disorder or the original majority population of cells being cultured [156, 198].

There is a report of two cell lines derived from HCL in which intranuclear herpes-type virus particles were found in most of the cells [346]; later work demonstrated that the virus produced by the cells from one of the lines was EBV of the African Burkitt's type, and that the cells were EBNA-positive [229]. However, it is possible that the EBV-producing cells were not derived from HCs, since the virus genome was not detectable in splenic HCs before culture and the cultured cells changed their SIg phenotype with time [229, 345].

It has been demonstrated that type 1 Herpes simplex virus can replicate in freshly isolated HCs, with the appearance of intranuclear virus particles [303]. It may be significant that, although HCs can support herpes virus replication, CLL cells that possess the EBV receptor do not allow Herpes simplex replication [303]. We are unable to comment on the significance of the intracisternal A-type virus particles noted in the plasma cells, but not the HCs, of a single case of HCL [289].

5.2.5 Receptors for Mouse Erythrocytes

The HCs of most cases of HCL have been reported to possess receptors for unsensitized mouse erythrocytes [67, 68, 322].

Spontaneous mouse erythrocyte (Mo) rosette formation has been shown to be a function of a small subpopulation of normal human B lymphocytes [162, 359]. For this reason the ability of HCs to form Mo rosettes is often cited as evidence for the B-lymphoid nature of HCL [344], although Mo receptor-negative cases have been reported [46, 67, 249].

We have studied 15 cases of HCL for this receptor. Seven never showed over 5% rosette formation by peripheral blood or splenic HCs, even on repeated testing. In the other eight patients, a mean of 14% of peripheral blood mononuclear cells expressed the receptor, while in the four of these cases in whom splenic cells were tested a rather higher mean percentage (34%) of splenic HCs formed Mo rosettes. This difference between peripheral blood and splenic mononuclear cells could not be attributed to contaminating T cells [46]. Analysis of the SIg phenotype of these 15 cases showed a correlation between Mo-receptor expression and the heavy-chain isotype. Thus, HCs expressing SIgG only did not form Mo rosettes, whereas in cases in which the cells had multiple heavy-chain isotypes at their surface the HCs also had Mo receptors [46].

Within the lymphoproliferative disorders, we and other investigators [22, 46, 67, 344] have found that significant Mo-rosette formation is restricted to the cells of HCL and CLL. Both this restriction and the demonstration that the Mo receptor appears early in normal B-cell ontogeny [163] suggest that the receptor is a marker of B cells early in their differentiation [344]. The finding that $SIgD^+$, but not $SIgG^+$, HCs express the Mo receptor lends further support to this suggestion, since $SIgG^+$ cells are probably more differentiated than those bearing multiple heavy-chain isotypes, including SIgD [55, 91, 138, 307].

5.2.6 Other Markers

Anti-hairy Cell Sera. Heteroantisera to HCs have been raised in rabbits by several groups [57, 213–215, 364]. Successful immunization has been achieved by means of 2 or 3 weekly iv injections of purified HCs from peripheral blood or spleen [57, 215].

Kitani [213–215] specifically absorbed the antiserum with normal leucocytes, B-CLL cells, or HCs, and tested the residual activity of these sera in a cytotoxic assay. Absorption with any of these cell types completely abolished killing of normal lymphocytes. HC killing was unaffected by absorption with normal leucocytes or CLL cells, but was removed by absorption with HCs. Cytotoxicity of B-CLL cells was maintained after absorption with normal leucocytes, but was abolished by absorption with either CLL cells or HCs. The lymph-node cells from four cases of "reticulum-cell sarcoma", including two T-cell cases, were also killed by the serum. This activity was unaffected by absorption with normal or CLL lymphocytes but was removed after absorption with HCs: a similar result was obtained from a single case of T-cell lymphosarcoma. Cells from two of four cases of null-cell ALL were specifically killed with the antiserum, but cells from T-cell ALL and the Sézary syndrome were uniformly negative. Leukaemic myeloid and monocytic cells from a variety of cases were invariably completely unreactive in the cytotoxic assay.

With our own sera, we have used a different approach involving immunofluorescence and progressive absorption, but have obtained essentially similar results. The original nonspecifically absorbed serum stained HCs from a variety of patients to a titre of 1/1,600. Progressive absorptions with a range of cell types were then carried out, and the reduction in titre following each absorption was noted. Absorptions were performed with cells from normal spleen and tonsil, and with cells from cases of the T-cell Sézary syndrome, chronic myeloid leukaemia, the acute monocytic leukaemias (both SCHILLING and NAEGELI types), and a myeloproliferative state with a large number of circulating normoblasts. There was some reduction in titre after each absorption, but no particular cell type caused a dramatic reduction. The serum was also absorbed with splenic cells from a case of Hodgkin's disease without significant loss in titre. This last absorption is of some interest, since there is a report of a virtually unabsorbed anti-HC serum, which did not stain T lymphocytes or myeloid cells, but was strongly positive with the Reed-Sternberg cells of Hodgkin's disease [364]. After these extensive absorptions, our serum completely failed to stain normal peripheral blood or splenic lymphocytes, erythrocytes or neutrophils, even when staining was carried out at a dilution of 1/5. The serum continued to stain HCs from most cases at 1/100, but it also stained CLL cells from some cases at a dilution of 1/10. Exhaustive absorption with CLL cells removed the anti-CLL activity, but the final activity of this serum against HCs was reduced to 1/10.

When this extensively absorbed serum was used in indirect staining techniques with peroxidase or ferritin labels and the stained cells were examined by electron microscopy [57], the complete surface of the HC showed immunochemical reaction product (Fig. 5.7). However, with very sensitive techniques such as immunoelectron microscopy it was noted that other cell types also showed some evidence of staining. It is probable that entirely monospecific heteroantisera can never be fully achieved by absorption, and that very sensitive techniques should probably be avoided. Nevertheless, in immunofluorescent tests employing the antiserum at the end of the plateau region of staining, the extensively absorbed serum appeared to be specific for HCs since other cell types, both normal and leukaemic, failed to stain. For this reason we have used the serum to estimate HC numbers within a given case of HCL and have generally found that the percentage of cells staining exceeded that of morphological HCs, but correlated with estimates of HC numbers by other methods (Table 5.2).

The absorbed anti-HC serum blocked the μFc receptor (and the apparent C3 receptor) on HCs to very high dilutions (100% inhibition consistently observed at 1/400). However, high concentrations of the serum (1/25) did not block E-rosette formation by normal T lymphocytes or by HCs with T-cell features (Sect. 5.6), nor did the serum block SIg., γFc-, or Mo-rosette formation by HCs. These blocking studies suggest that the antigen being detected by the anti-HC serum is either the μFc receptor itself or a closely adjacent structure. The opinion that the blocking is due to steric hindrance is supported by the fact that the μFc receptor on CLL cells was only partially blocked by high concentrations (1/10) of this antiserum.

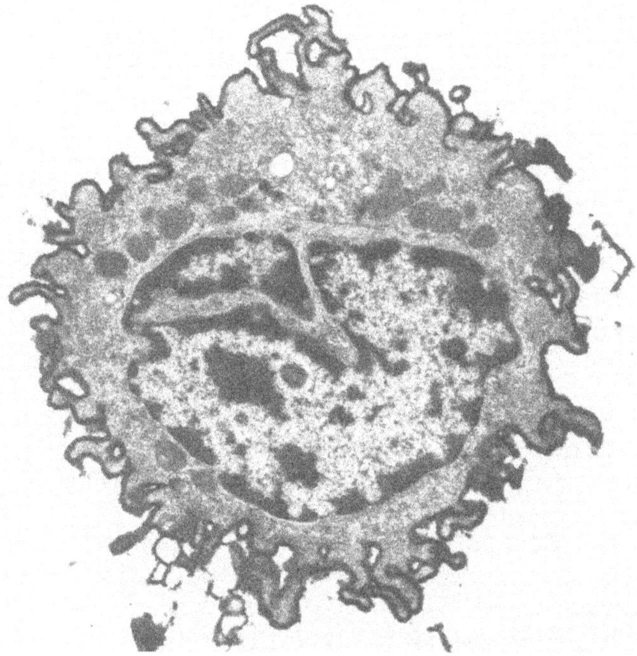

Fig. 5.7. Immunoperoxidase staining of an HC with an anti-HC serum. Strong reaction product coats the entire cell surface (× 10,000)

Table 5.2. Staining of HCs with an anti-HC serum[a] and the correlation with other surface markers

Patient	Morphological HCs %	Anti-HC staining %	T cells %	γFc %	SIg %
DC	5	23	83	12	8
AD	60	80	18	82	66
PS	35	73	42	73	62
LH	33	68	33	77	70

[a] Fc binding was avoided by the use of recently ultracentrifuged serum for viable cells and by the use of acetone-fixed cells

Ia-like Antigen and Other Surface Glycoproteins. HCs express the HLA-D-related antigen complex that is the human counterpart of the mouse Ia antigen [54, 77, 270, 272, 328]. Hairy cells have been examined with absorbed alloantisera specific for the HLA-D-related group [270, 272, 328] and with heteroantisera raised to the purified glycoprotein complex [54, 77]. We have studied splenic and peripheral blood mononuclear cells from six cases of HCL with a monospecific heteroantiserum to the glycoprotein complex (p29, 34) [355] in an indirect fluorescent technique. In all cases, virtually all the cells that were not T lymphocytes stained strongly. Blocking studies with this antiserum, and the possible significance of the presence of the Ia-like antigen on HCs, will be discussed below (Sect. 5.3).

Various cell populations, both normal and leukaemic, have been studied for surface glycoproteins, and characteristic profiles have been established [10, 11]. Hairy cells display a

distinctive glycoprotein profile resembling that of B-lymphoblastoid cell lines, but quite different from that of CLL cells and of normal and leukaemic monocytes [9].
The nature and function of most of the surface glycoproteins of haemic cells are not known, but two functionally important proteins have been identified at bands corresponding to molecular weights of 24,000 and 31,000, and of 210,000; these are subunits of the Ia-like antigen and fibronectin respectively. Hairy cells have a prominent band in the GP 24,31 region [9], and this correlates well with the strong staining reaction obtained with anti-Ia-like antisera. Fibronectin, which is probably a dimeric form of GP210, has attracted considerable attention recently because of its importance in substrate adherence (reviewed in [12]). Fibronectin is present on human monocytes and B lymphocytes (both normal and leukaemic), but not on granulocytes or T lymphocytes [10, 133]. Despite their glass-adherent properties (Sect. 5.3.2), HCs do not have GP210 as a dominant surface glycoprotein [9] and do not stain with specific anti-fibronectin antisera [9].

Monkey Erythrocyte Rosettes. HCs form spontaneous rosettes with monkey erythrocytes (Mk) obtained from Rhesus and Cynomorgus monkeys.
The formation of spontaneous Mk rosettes by human leucocytes has been described as a specific marker both for T cells [242] and for B lymphocytes and B-lymphoblastoid cell lines [120, 290]. However, we have observed Mk-rosette formation by a variety of human leukaemic cells, regardless of the cell lineage, and have demonstrated that Mk rosettes are formed between complement components on the leucocyte membrane and the immune adherence receptor present on Mk [45]. We have examined peripheral blood mononuclear cells from 20 cases of HCL and have found that the majority of HCs invariably form Mk rosettes, and that in some cases a proportion of the T lymphocytes present also form rosettes. Hairy cells form strong Mk rosettes, often with ten or more erythrocytes attached (Fig. 5.8), and these are not readily disrupted mechanically.
The method of complement deposition on the HC membrane is unknown, but several mechanisms can be envisaged. Many leukaemias elicit autoantibody, perhaps against a tumour-associated antigen [59], and it has been suggested that there is autoantibody on the surface of some cases of HCL [13]; this might lead to direct complement activation at the cell membrane. Alternatively, Fc binding of immune complexes, formed either from autoantibody or as a result of recent infections, could lead to complement being associated with the cell membrane. In this context, a recent report of a case of HCL with polyarteritis nodosa [183], in which circulating immune complexes were demonstrated, is of interest. However, HCs themselves may manufacture the complement on the surface membrane, since the HCs from a primary culture maintained in complement-free medium for several weeks formed over 90% Mk rosettes [45].
Whatever the mechanism, the high rate of Mk-rosette formation seen in HCL contrasts with the generally low percentage of rosette formation usually seen in CLL [45], and Mk-rosette formation provides a useful additional diagnostic test for HCL.

Human Erythrocyte Rosettes. Spontaneous autorosette formation with human erythrocytes is probably a marker for thymocytes [344]; HCs are negative for this receptor [45].

Cholera Toxin-binding Sites. Two cases of HCL have been tested for the presence of the monosialoganglioside molecule (GMI), which is the high-affinity surface receptor for cholergen, the active protein component of cholera toxin. The cells from both cases were reported to lack the GMI receptor [309]. This was an unexpected and unexplained result since, apart from

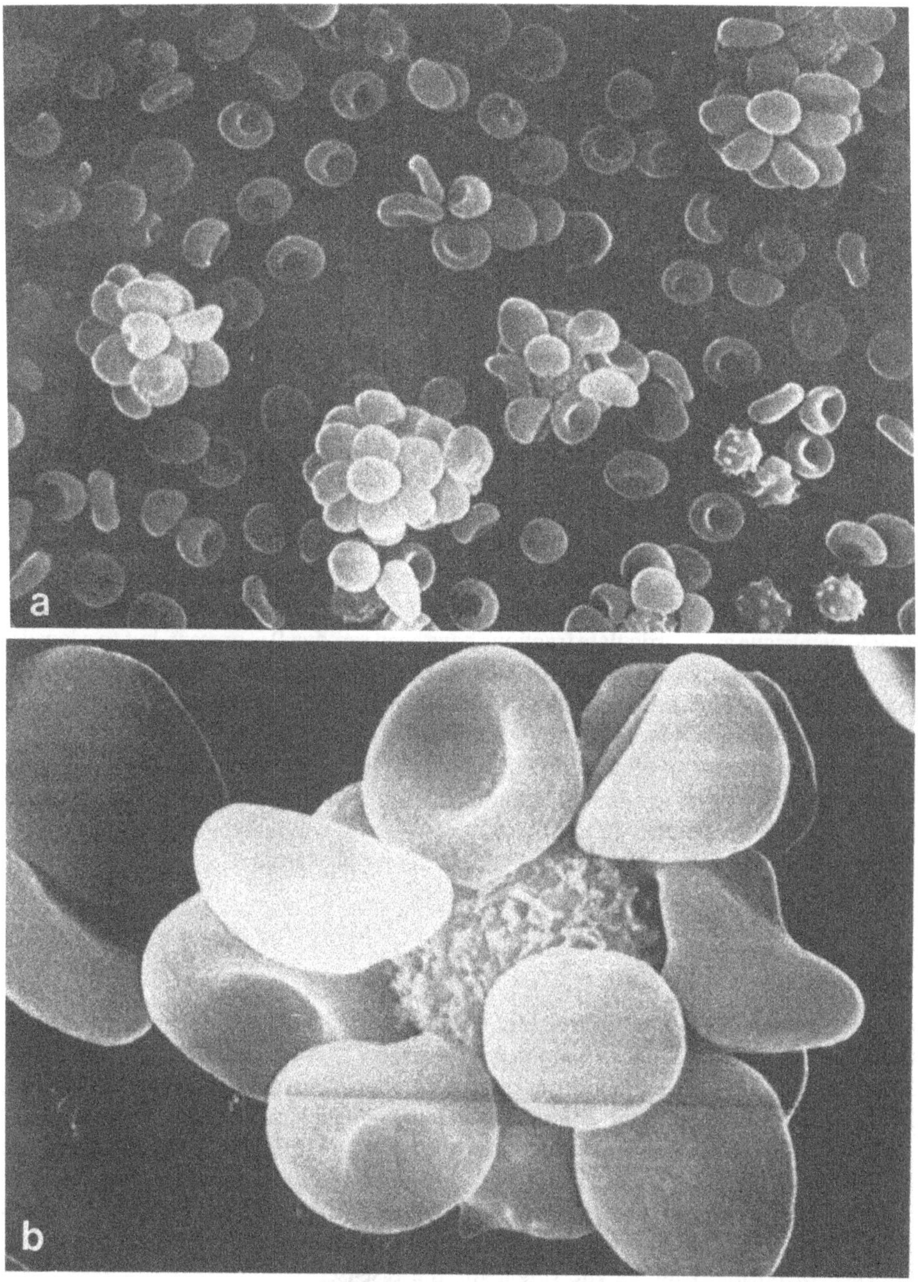

Fig. 5.8a, b. Scanning electron microscopy of HCs forming Mk rosettes. The large rosettes involve many firmly attached indicator cells. The Mk erythrocytes are not deformed, and in **b** are seen to make point contact mainly with the surface microvilli (**a** × 2,500; **b** × 10,000)

erythroid cells, most normal human haemic cells express the receptor, and among the leukaemias only acute leukaemias are negative [309]. In the same report, 11 cases of CLL showed strong cholera-toxin labelling, and it was suggested that glycolipid changes were linked with the malignant process and that cholera-toxin binding served as a marker distinguishing acute from chronic leukaemic cells. However, since in many cell types the cholera-toxin receptor can be exposed by neuraminidase treatment, it may be that GMI expression is not directly related to cell type, but rather to sialic acid masking the GMI receptor to a greater or less extent. Alternatively, since normal human and mouse myeloma plasma cells fail to bind cholera toxin [87, 309], it may be that this receptor is lost during the later stages of B-cell development.

Lectin-binding Sites. Limited lectin-binding studies have shown that HCs bind most lectins (PHA, concanavalin A, wheat germ agglutinin, Ricinis communis agglutinin) in greater amounts than other lymphocyte types [27]. The significance of these findings is not clear, although it has been suggested that concanavalin A binding may be the result of pinocytosis [322].

Steroid Receptors. HCs possess specific binding sites for prednisone and, to a lesser extent, for dexamethasone [15]. Whole-cell uptake of these steroids is greater for HCs than for CLL cells, but this may simply reflect relative cell size. Steroid binding by solubilized material (from which membrane and particulate fractions have been removed) is present, but to a low degree, in both HCL and CLL cells. When such cytosol finding is expressed in terms of unit volume of cytoplasm, HCs bind relatively less prednisolone than CLL cells, and virtually no dexamethasone [15].

The in vitro sensitivity of HCL and CLL cells to methyl prednisolone has been measured and compared [15]. For up to 120 h of culture, HCs are resistant to killing by concentrations as high as 10^{-4} *M*. In contrast, CLL cells show dose-related cell death, a high percentage of non-viable cells being found at 10^{-4} *M* concentrations of steroid.

5.3 Monocytic Features

Hairy cells possess a number of features usually associated with monocytes, and this has led some authors to define HCL as a monocytic disorder [13, 104, 185, 199, 211, 285, 286, 302, 312, 322, 333, 342]. Such monocytic features include: adherence to glass and plastic [27, 69, 316]; retention by nylon fibre columns [27, 389]; phagocytosis of latex particles [93, 129, 166, 395]; possession of strong receptors for the Fc of IgG (γFc) [182, 185, 211]; presence of NSE enzymes [199, 322]; and surface ruffles on SEM [302]. In addition to these "monocytic features" of HCs, the absence of normal monocytes in the peripheral blood of patients with HCL [342] and the peculiar reticuloendothelial distribution of HCs [104] constitute indirect evidence favouring a monocytic origin for the disease.

However, there is agreement that several important monocytic features are absent. Thus, HCs do not develop into typical macrophages on short-term culture [43, 58, 69, 144, 286, 308, 331, 339], although an increase in cytoplasmic granules has been noted after short periods of in vitro culture [286]. HCs do not contain or produce lysozyme [43, 64, 329, 335, 397], and do not possess peroxidase-positive granules at any stage of their development [312]. In addition, typical HCs, unlike both normal and leukaemic monocytes, do not produce colony-stimulating factor (CSF) when used as a feeder layer for normal bone-marrow cells

[141, 169, 350, 365, 395], although there is a report of cultured T-cell HCs producing CSF [142].

In the present section, we consider the alleged monocytic features of HCs and conclude that many are compatible with a lymphoid origin for the HC.

5.3.1 Morphological Aspects

Cytology and Cytochemistry. In ROMANOWSKY preparations HCs do not resemble monocytes, but early studies of HCL paid particular attention to the phase-contrast appearances of HCs, comparing them with monocytes and lymphocytes [29, 258, 308, 325, 339, 372, 389]. These studies showed variable flattening on glass and cytoplasmic movement, particularly when examined by time-lapse microcinematography [372] – findings that seemed perhaps to relate HCs more to monocytes than lymphocytes. Nevertheless, most of the authors concerned [29, 308, 339, 372, 389] concluded that HCs differed from both cell types.

The same is true of the cytochemistry of HCs. In particular, NSE staining of HCs, which has been cited as a monocytic feature [199, 258, 322], gives a distinctive staining pattern [177] different from that of both monocytes and lymphocytes; and, unlike monocytic esterase, HC staining is not inhibited by sodium fluoride [177, 335, 373].

Hairy cells have recently been shown to possess a peroxidase activity, distinct from myeloperoxidase, in their endoplasmic reticulum and perinuclear cistern (Sect. 4.3.1). Since this peroxidase activity is absent from B and T lymphocytes, but present in monocytes and macrophages, it has been cited as evidence favouring a monocytic origin for HCs [312]. However, this argument is weakened by the fact that a similar peroxidatic activity is present in platelets [34].

Ultrastructure. None of the TEM features of HCs specifically relates them to either monocytes or lymphocytes, and we concur with DANIEL and FLANDRIN [93], who conclude that the ultrastructure of HCs is characteristic and distinctive. In contrast, the surface ruffles frequently seen on HCs by SEM (Fig. 4.27) do seem to be a monocytic feature, since they are rarely observed on lymphoid cells [33, 301]. These surface ruffles are one of the most difficult monocytic features of HCs to reconcile with a lymphoid nature. However, since the surface topography of minor subpopulations of lymphocytes is largely unknown, it may be that surface ruffles are not strictly confined to monocytic cells.

5.3.2 Adhesive Properties and Phagocytosis

Hairy cells are sticky cells and tend to clump together and adhere strongly to a variety of surfaces. For example, although there have been reports to the contrary [249, 322, 372], glass and plastic adherence is the experience of most workers [27, 44, 69, 101, 211, 286, 316]. Although there are reports of cases of HCL showing that HCs pass through nylon fibre columns [325, 361], other groups [27, 68, 96, 375] have found that HCs are retained. We have shown [44] that HCs were also retained by a sephadex G-10 column, which is generally considered to remove monocytes [4, 245]. However, these techniques probably also remove some B lymphocytes, particularly those cells bearing SIg of IgG or IgA type [4] – SIg isotypes frequently expressed by HCs [56, 191]. The HCs were not eluted from the G-10 column with EDTA [44], and this observation is in accord with that of RIEBER et al. [316], who have shown that glass-adherent HCs are more resistant than monocytes to removal by EDTA-trypsin treatment. The nonspecific stickiness of HCs in almost all manipulations is probably at least partly a consequence of the complex nature of their surface structure (reviewed by LOOR [243]).

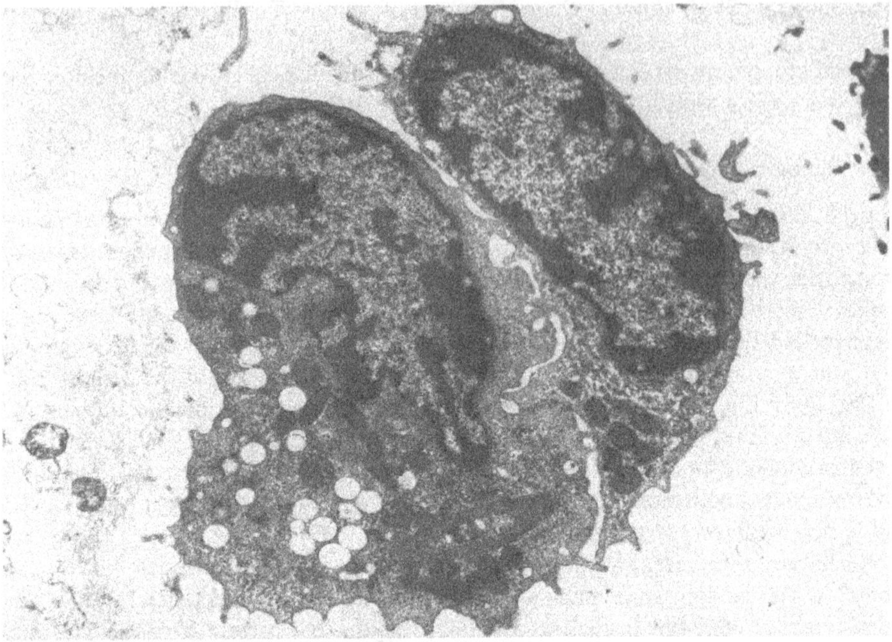

Fig. 5.9. Phagocytosis of latex particles. Both the HCs contain internalized latex particles. One of the HCs is unequivocally identified by the presence of three R-L complexes (× 9,500)

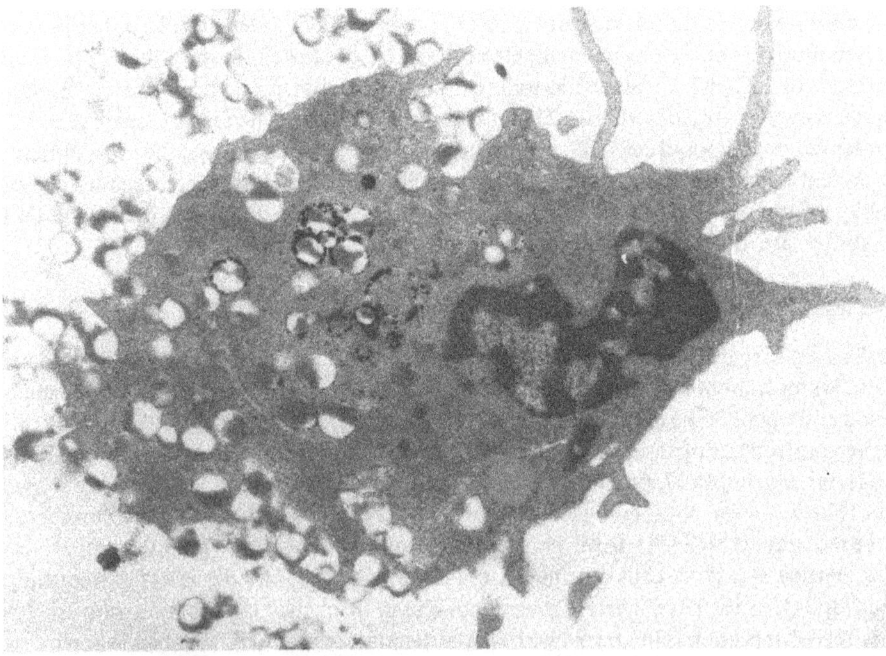

Fig. 5.10. Latex phagocytosis and acid-phosphatase cytochemistry. The presence of acid phosphatase reaction product around many of the latex particles indicates that they are truly phagocytosed. Lead citrate staining only (× 14,000)

Therefore, it can reasonably be argued that all their adherence features are compatible with the view that HCs are lymphocytes with a complex surface topography [243].

The same arguments can be employed to explain the phagocytosis of latex particles. With few exceptions [249, 339, 389], there is almost complete agreement that HCs can phagocytose latex [27, 69, 93, 129, 166, 191, 211, 286, 322, 375, 395], and we can confirm this since we have observed latex phagocytosis in all of ten cases of HCL examined (> 80% of HCs contained latex by TEM) (Fig. 5.9). There is less agreement about phagocytosis of anything other than latex. In most reports, carbon black, yeast, and bacteria, whether opsonized or not, are not phagocytosed by HCs [21, 101, 129, 164, 211, 213, 325, 389], and JANSEN et al. [191, 192] demonstrated with lysostaphin that apparently phagocytosed staphylococci were cell-associated rather than internalized. While confirming that HCs are not effectively phagocytic for yeast or opsonized erythrocytes, we have established that latex particles are truly phagocytosed, since ultrastructural acid-phosphatase cytochemistry demonstrated the release of this enzyme into a proportion of the phagocytic vacuoles [44] (Fig. 5.10). However, despite this demonstration, the poor phagocytosis of anything but latex suggests that HCs are not professional phagocytes. In any event, phagocytosis is not a property exclusive to the monocyte-macrophage series, since the B cells of CLL [71, 395] and a variety of other cells, including T cells bearing a γFc receptor, are capable of phagocytosis [127, 161]. In these instances, as in phagocytosis by HCs, it is probably the attachment phase that is the determining event for subsequent internalization; this attachment is enhanced in HCL by the inherent stickiness of the cells.

5.3.3 γFc Receptors and the Ia Antigen

The possession of a strong receptor for the Fc of IgG (γFcR) is one of the features of HCs that have led to the suggestion that these cells belong to the monocyte-histiocyte series [185, 211, 333]. Indeed, in many features the γFc receptor of HCs does resemble that on monocytes rather than that on most normal SIg-positive B lymphocytes: some of these points of comparison are summarized in Table 5.3. Nevertheless, as is seen in Table 5.3, many of the monocyte-type γFcR characteristics are also possessed by an unclassified cell group (UCG) variously described in man as third-population cells [128], null cells [83], K cells [291], and L cells [179]. Although these unclassified cells are probably heterogeneous in terms of their surface phenotype and potential functions [178, 334], some are Ia-positive [334] and can differentiate to synthesize and secrete immunoglobulin [82]. Therefore, in view of the undoubted immunoglobulin production by HCs, the "monocytoid" features of their γFc receptor seem to relate them more closely to this UCG group than to monocytes.

5.3.4 Monocytopenia and Reticuloendothelial Distribution

The suggestion that the almost complete peripheral blood monocytopenia in HCL [57, 177, 189, 342, 373, 385] favours a monocytic origin for HCs [342] is considerably weakened by the fact that splenic and bone-marrow macrophages and Kupffer cells, which derive from blood monocytes [103], are usually plentiful in the disease [33, 153, 274; Chap. 3], while HCs have never been shown to transform into macrophages. The reason for the peripheral monocytopenia of the disease therefore remains uncertain, and for further discussion of this point the reader is referred to Chap. 6.

The explanation of the distinctive reticuloendothelial distribution of HCs [104, 361] will remain obscure until further work is done on the various factors influencing cell migration.

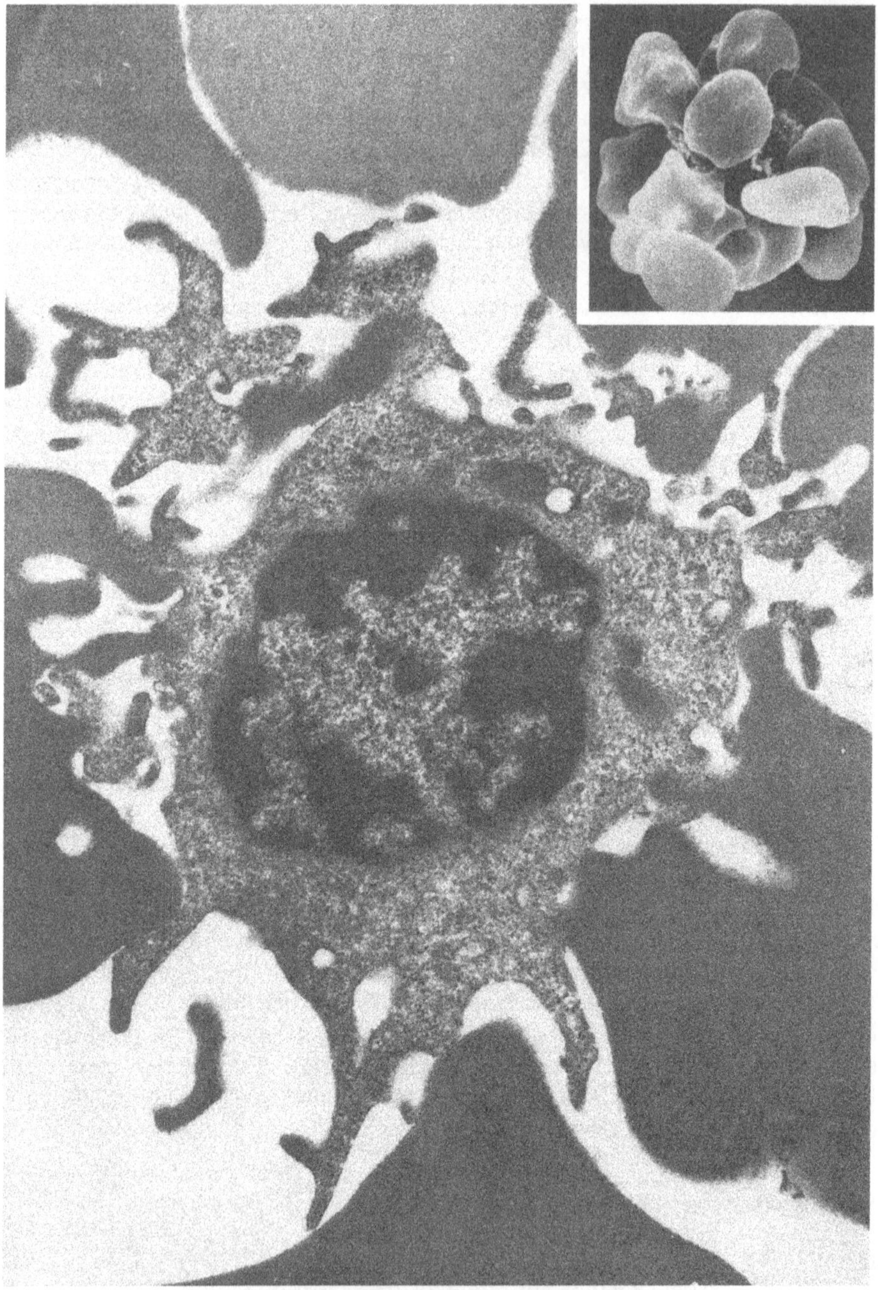

Fig. 5.11. Morphology of γFc rosettes formed by HCs. Many indicator erythrocytes are involved in the rosette. These make contact with the HCs over large areas of its surface and are markedly deformed in the process (TEM × 15,000; *inset* SEM × 4,000)

Table 5.3. Comparison of the γFc receptor on monocytes and UCG[a] cells, on B lymphocytes, and on HCs

Test	Monocytes and UCG	B lympho-cytes	HCs	References
EAG-rosette formation with erythrocytes coated with < 5,000 IgG molecules (e.g., with anti-Rh or anti-Forssman antibodies)	+	–	+	44, 185, 211, 238, 278, 343
Deformation of sensitized erythrocytes forming rosettes	+	–	+	47, 240, 288; Fig. 5.11
Binding of EAG by frozen sections of tissue and/or by glass-adherent monolayers	+	–	+	44, 102, 191, 211, 249, 343
Receptor sensitive to protease	–	+	–	106, 249
Receptor blocked by anti-Ia-like antigen[b]	–	+	–	44, 107, 108, 334, 351

[a] Unclassified cell group includes null cells, K cells, third-population cells, and L cells (see text)
[b] Blocking of EAG-rosette formation, but not of antibody-mediated cell cytotoxicity

However, since both surface markers and surface topography are known to influence the migratory properties of cells [243, 353], it is possible to speculate that the unique immunological phenotype and the distinctive surface ruffles of HCs are important factors in determining their distribution.

5.4 Immunoglobulin Synthesis and Secretion

The weight of evidence suggests that, in addition to synthesizing SIg, HCs secrete Ig, usually with an excess of free light chains. Analysis of supernatants from HC cultures has shown Ig synthesis and secretion, and immunofluorescence studies have proved that the Ig is produced by the HC and is not a product of contaminating plasma cells.

5.4.1 Immunoglobulin Secretion

Newly synthesized Ig has been demonstrated in the supernatant of cultured HCs by immunoprecipitation of radiolabelled protein [80, 144, 154, 315, 325, 331] and by a microagglutination method [58, 80]. The main classes secreted are IgG and IgM [58, 80, 325, 331], although IgD has been found [155]. GORDON and SMITH [154, 155] have shown that, irrespective of the heavy-chain class being synthesized, and even in a SIg-negative case, HCs secrete a great excess of free light chains. Others [315] have also observed excess light-chain secretion in HCL – a phenomenon that is a feature of several B-cell neoplasms, including CLL [156, 246]. Predominant free light-chain secretion may account for the report that the cells from a single case of HCL did not produce IgG, IgM or IgA, even when cultured in the presence of PWM [33].

5.4.2 Cytoplasmic Immunoglobulin

Cells expressing SIg but not secreting Ig (for example, CLL lymphocytes) are usually negative for intracytoplasmic Ig (CIg) [305]. The demonstration that HCs synthesize CIg of restricted light-chain type [58, 144, 154, 164, 191, 361, 375, 395] therefore suggests that it is these cells which secrete the Ig detected in culture experiments. Intracytoplasmic Ig in HCs has been demonstrated by immunofluorescence [58, 144, 164, 191, 350, 395] and by immunoprecipitation of lysates of cells cultured in the presence of radiolabelled amino acids [88, 154]. The main isotypes detected have been IgG and IgM, although there have been reports of cases with CIgD [58, 395], CIgA [164], and light chain alone [58]. However, in some cases the HCs completely lack CIg [33, 191], and in positive cases the intensity of fluorescence is never as strong as that seen in plasma cells.

5.4.3 Paraproteinaemia

On rare occasions HCL may be associated with paraproteinaemia [80, 112, 143, 315], and in some instances it has been possible to show that the pathological cells probably produced the paraprotein [80, 143].

We have reported a case of HCL with IgGk paraproteinaemia, in which it was demonstrated that the HCs were synthesizing IgGk, as evidenced by cytoplasmic staining, SIg re-expression following stripping, and the analysis (by microagglutination and radioimmunoprecipitation) of the supernatant of cultured cells [80]. Apart from the presence of paraproteinaemia, this case was clinically, haematologically, cytologically and immunologically entirely typical.

There was no excess of plasma cells, no lytic bone lesions, no Bence-Jones proteinuria and no immuneparesis. The paraprotein was present in only small amounts (6 g/litre) and did not increase over a prolonged period. Recently, we have been informed of another case of typical HCL with IgGk paraproteinaemia [212]. There has also been a report of HCL with transient IgGλ cryocrystalglobulinaemia; in this patient the HCs possessed intracytoplasmic IgGλ, but no paraproteinaemia was detectable [220].

GOLDE et al. [143] described a case of HCL with an IgM paraprotein, but the patient's disease was atypical in a number of respects [80] and the diagnosis has been questioned [13, 210]. We cannot comment on the significance of the IgM paraproteinaemia present in one of the cases reported by RIEBER et al. [315], since these authors were careful to point out that, despite thorough investigation, they could not demonstrate IgM synthesis by the HCs.

It is difficult to account for the rarity of paraproteinaemia and Bence-Jones proteinuria in HCL, particularly since the HCs from many cases secrete Ig and have readily detectable CIg – a feature only seen in CLL cells when the patient has a paraprotein [305]. It is also difficult to understand why our patient has a paraprotein, since both the light-to-heavy chain imbalance and the rate of in vitro synthesis of Ig by his HCs were similar to those of HCs from several other cases without paraproteinaemia [80]. Furthermore, there was no detectable plasmacytosis in the patient and his HCs showed no evidence of plasmacytoid differentiation. The explanation for the occasional paraproteinaemia in the disease must, therefore, remain obscure; but while an undetected plasmacytosis can never be entirely excluded, it is possible to speculate either that the half-life of the Ig subclass plays a part or that T-cell help may be greater in these rare cases.

Plasma cells are often conspicuous in a variety of tissues from cases of HCL without paraproteinaemia. Immunoperoxidase [153, 279] and immunofluorescence studies [33] have demonstrated that these plasma cells are not involved in the monoclonal proliferation. Moreover, ultrastructural studies have found no plasmacytoid differentiation by HCs and no R-L complexes in the plasma cells [153], although these complexes have been reported in myeloma plasma cells [37, 159]. The plentiful tissue plasma cells are compatible with the lack of immuneparesis characteristic of the disease [153].

5.5 Summary of the Immunological Membrane Phenotype of Typical HCs

The purpose of this section is briefly to outline the more important surface-marker characteristics of HCs presented in detail in this chapter. This is done to provide a summary of earlier sections of the chapter, to give some indication of how immunological markers may be of diagnostic value, and to enable easier reading of Sect. 5.6 which describes the complex nature of T-cell cases of HCL and assumes familiarity with abbreviated immunological marker terminology.

Hairy cells are almost invariably positive for receptors for the Fc of IgG (γFc), but this is a ubiquitous marker present on most haemic cell types. A proportion of HCs usually bear receptors for the Fc of IgM (μFc), and these are detectable without prior culture. The cells must be tested rapidly after separation and, in the rosette test employed, high levels of sensitizing IgM antibody must be used. The presence of a μFc receptor demonstrable without culture distinguishes HCs from most lymphoma and leukaemia cells, except those of CLL. Monoclonal SIg is usually present on typical HCs. The density is greater than that seen on most CLL cells, but more characteristic is the distribution of heavy-chain isotypes. Some 50% of cases of HCL have HCs bearing SIgG only, and the rest have cells with multiple heavy-chain isotypes.

The frequency of the isotypes present in the multiple cases is distinctive, with IgD, IgG, and/or IgA usually exceeding IgM; this is in contrast to most CLL cells, where IgM and IgD are usually prominent. There are, however, cases of IgG-only CLL, prolymphocytic leukaemia, and non-Hodgkin's lymphoma. The HCs from most cases of HCL do not form sheep erythrocyte (E) rosettes.

Thus the marker profile of typical HCs is $\gamma Fc^{+}\mu Fc^{+}SIg^{+}E^{-}$.

Other immunological markers we have found useful in identifying HCs are receptors for mouse erythrocytes (Mo) and for rhesus monkey erythrocytes (Mk), and the general absence of receptors for the fixed component of complement (C3). High spontaneous Mo-rosette formation is not usually seen in HCL, although a low percentage is frequently observed; high Mo will usually suggest CLL. Conversely, high Mk can often exclude CLL and prolymphocytic leukaemia, although high Mk is not confined to HCL. The absence of the C3 receptor helps in differentiating HCL from many B-cell lymphomas and, if reagents detecting C3d are used, from CLL.

5.6 T-cell Features

Several cases of HCL with T-cell features have now been described [1, 48, 54, 77, 79, 174, 190, 272, 330]. In all these cases, morphologically typical HCs formed spontaneous rosettes with sheep erythrocytes. With the possible exceptions of skin rash and pruritus in one patient [174] and the development of high leucocyte counts after splenectomy in two [190], none of the T-cell cases had unusual clinical or haematological features.

Two of the cases described were studied with only a limited panel of immunological markers [1, 174], and the recorded cell phenotypes for the cases were $E^{+}\gamma Fc^{-}C3^{-}$ [1] and $E^{+}C3^{-}$ [174].

Saxon et al. [330] investigated their case extensively with a variety of markers and found that the cells both formed E rosettes and reacted with a specifically absorbed, heterologous, anti-T cell serum (anti-T). The cells did not express γFc or C3 receptors and did not possess SIg or CIg. Radiolabelling studies demonstrated that the cells did not synthesize immunoglobulin in vitro. The case tested by Naeim et al. [272] was also $E^{+}SIg^{-}\gamma Fc^{-}C3^{-}$. The last-named authors also tested the cells with alloantisera to the Ia-like antigens and found them (in contrast to typical HCs) to be negative; however, these cells were able to stimulate in mixed lymphocyte cultures.

Cases of HCL with T-cell features, but with a completely different phenotypic profile, have been observed both in our own studies [48, 54, 77] and by Jansen et al. [190]. These cases differed slightly in their precise marker characteristics, but all had the true T-B hybrid phenotype $E^{+}SIg^{+}$. Extensive investigations excluded technical artifact as the reason for this unusual phenotype. The detailed phenotype of the HCs in each of the four cases was as follows: E^{+}anti-$T^{+}SIg^{+}CIg^{+}Ia^{+}\gamma Fc^{+}\mu Fc^{+}Mo^{+}C3^{-}EBNA^{-}$ [77]; $E^{+}SIg^{+}CIg^{+}\gamma Fc^{+}\mu Fc^{+}C3^{-}$ [79] (the cells also secreted Ig); E^{+}anti-$T^{+}SIg^{+}CIg^{+}$ [190]; E^{+}anti-$T^{+}SIg^{+}CIg^{+}Ia^{-}\gamma Fc^{+}\mu Fc^{+}Mo^{+}C3^{-}TdT^{-}$ [190].

Jansen et al. [190] considered that such T-B hybrid cases represented a distinct subtype of HCL, but sequential marker studies [48, 79] make it clear that this is not so. Follow-up studies of both our hybrid cases [48] showed that wide variations in the marker phenotype of the HCs occurred; and, if either case had been studied on a single occasion, very different interpretations of the basic cell type could have been made. Thus, at various times, either case could have been considered a typical case of B-cell HCL ($E^{-}SIg^{+}\gamma Fc^{+}C3^{-}$), or one patient

could have been described as a case of "pure" (E^+SIg^-) T-cell HCL. One of the cases described by JANSEN et al. [190] was followed for some 2 months, and changed in phenotype from a predominantly E^+ anti-T^+ cell with some SIg to a predominantly SIg^+ cell that formed some E rosettes. These results emphasize the importance of using a panel of markers for the characterization of lymphoproliferative disorders [36, 54, 306] and the necessity for sequential studies [99, 181], particularly in cases described as unusual.
Further phenotypic variations were observed in these hybrid cases when different tissues were examined. For example, at a time when the peripheral blood cells displayed T-cell features, the splenic cells from both the cases described by JANSEN et al. [190] had the B-cell phenotype E^-anti-$T^-SIg^+\gamma Fc^+$. We have recently observed two cases of typical HCL with the usual peripheral blood phenotype of $E^-SIg^+\gamma Fc^+$, which had a high proportion of morphologically typical HCs in the spleen with the phenotype E^+SIg^-. In our own reported hybrid cases, one had distinctly hybrid cells in the spleen but later, when the peripheral blood cells were predominantly E^+SIg^-, morphological HCs in the bone marrow were also E^+SIg^- [48]. The splenic HCs from our other case were predominantly E^-SIg^+, but the peripheral blood cells also had this phenotype at the time of splenectomy [48]. These cases argue against the hypothesis [190] that the spleen selectively sequesters HCs with a B-cell phenotype. Moreover, the splenic HCs of both the cases described by JANSEN et al. [190], although displaying the typical B-cell phenotype $E^-SIg^+\gamma Fc^+$, were unusual in that these cells were negative for the Ia-like antigen.
Some typical cases of HCL enter a phase in which circulating morphological HCs disappear, to be replaced by E-rosetting cells of lymphoid appearance (Sect. 2.6.2). These T lymphocytes are abnormal in a number of respects and may be involved in the clonal proliferation [76]. The existence of hybrid T-B cases, which can fluctuate widely, raises the possibility that typical morphological HCs with the characteristic $E^-SIg^+\gamma Fc^+$ B-cell phenotype can become $E^+SIg^-\gamma Fc^-$ lymphoid cells. There is no direct evidence to support this possibility, but two observations may be relevant. In one of our T-B hybrid cases, early in the E^+SIg^- phase some peripheral blood cells of lymphoid morphology possessed the R-L complex [48]; at the same time, some E^+SIg^- cells in the bone marrow had a typical HC morphology.

6 Other Haemic Cells

6.1 Granulocytes

6.1.1 Neutrophils

The quantitative neutrophil deficiency that is often present in HCL has been considered in Chap. 2. In addition, however, there are a number of features that suggest a qualitative neutrophil defect. The neutrophils consistently display an elevated level of alkaline phosphatase activity (Fig. 6.1), and the leukocyte alkaline phosphatase (LAP) score is almost always greater than 150 [171, 189, 202, 322]. Since elevated LAP scores are characteristic of myelofibrosis, the high score of HCL may be related to the marrow fibrosis of the disease; but this is not necessarily so, because high scores are also sometimes found in CLL [170]. Also, we have observed that in some patients the neutrophils fail to stain with either Sudan black or peroxidase methods: this abnormality may or may not be related to the neutrophil hypogranularity occasionally noted at the ultrastructural level.

The neutrophils of most cases of HCL are also functionally abnormal. Skin-window studies have shown that neutrophil migration to the site of inflammation is suboptimal, and neutrophil mobilization following iv hydrocortisone is markedly abnormal [385]. In addition, we have demonstrated defective intracellular candidacidal activity in eight of ten patients studied, and reduced staphylococcal killing in five of these cases [84]. In the three cases studied before and after splenectomy, an improvement in neutrophil function followed this procedure [84].

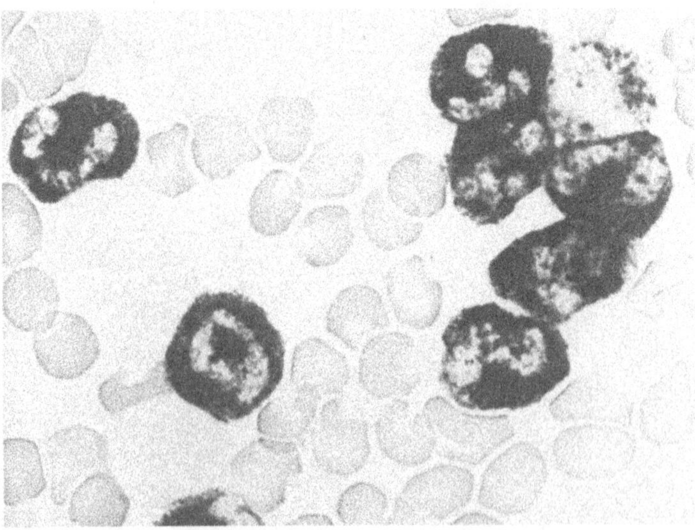

Fig. 6.1. The high neutrophil alkaline phosphatase score of HCL. This area of the buffy coat preparation shows the intense enzyme activity characteristically present in the neutrophils

The cause of the various qualitative defects in the neutrophils of HCL is not clear. Splenomegaly cannot play a primary aetiological role, since neutrophil defects are sometimes observed in patients who have previously undergone splenectomy [84, 385]. However, the improved neutrophil function sometimes observed after removal of the spleen indicates some splenic effect and provides further justification for therapeutic splenectomy. Since qualitative neutrophil defects are also seen in a wide variety of conditions involving invasion or fibrosis of the bone marrow [35, 85, 98, 113], it seems that marrow replacement rather than direct stem-cell involvement is a possible explanation of the qualitative neutrophil abnormalities of HCL [84, 385]. But, since eosinophils are not depressed in the disease, humoral inhibition of the granulocyte-macrophage progenitor is another possible explanation of both quantitative and qualitative neutrophil defects.

6.1.2 Eosinophils and Basophils

Unlike neutrophils and monocytes, eosinophils and basophils are not consistently reduced in the peripheral blood of HCL patients. This observation probably has some significance, since in vitro colony growth experiments have shown that neutrophils and monocytes share a common progenitor, while eosinophils develop independently [257]. It is likely, therefore, that the neutropenia and monocytopenia of HCL are attributable not only to marrow invasion but to humoral inhibitory factors specific for the neutrophil-macrophage progenitor. Such humoral factors might well be produced by HCs themselves, although it has been reported that HCs do not influence haematopoiesis in in vivo diffusion chamber experiments [369]. Nothing is known about the functional capacity of eosinophils and basophils in the disease.

6.2 Monocytes

There is wide agreement that HCL is characterized by an almost complete monocytopenia in the peripheral blood [31, 53, 57, 177, 189, 342, 373, 385], although occasional cases of HCL with significant numbers of monocytes continue to be reported [151]. In our experience, all typical cases have shown severe monocytopenia in both peripheral blood ($0–0.025 \times 10^9$/litre) and bone marrow, but in two atypical patients (Sect. 7.2) monocytopenia was not present (monocytes: $0.4–0.5 \times 10^9$/litre). The monocytopenia of our typical cases was confirmed by NSE staining and by careful examination of a mononuclear cell preparation at the ultrastructural level; the very occasional monocytes observed with TEM were of normal morphology. In contrast, the monocytes present in one of the atypical cases contained numerous large, abnormal granules (Fig. 7.5).
Despite the normal appearance of the few monocytes present in the peripheral blood of typical cases of HCL and the fact that these differentiate into macrophages on culture, there is evidence from skin-window studies that they show deficient migration [335, 342, 385]. This is not simply attributable to peripheral monocytopenia, for defective monocyte migration is not observed in non-Hodgkin's lymphoma with comparable monocytopenia [385]. Moreover, in vitro studies [216, 373] have shown that the serum of HCL patients contains a factor that inhibits chemotaxis of normal monocytes and neutrophils.
It is difficult to reconcile the monocytopenia of HCL with the fact that phagocytic reticuloendothelial cells are frequently abundant in the spleen, liver, and bone marrow of patients with the disease [33, 274; see also Chap. 3]. Hairy cells do not develop into macrophages in

culture (Sect. 4.7) and very few monocytes or monocyte precursors are observed in the bone marrow. Perhaps the most likely explanation is that some tissue macrophages are not derived from monocytes and are self-perpetuating.

6.3 Platelets

Thrombocytopenia is one of the most consistent findings in HCL (Chap. 2). There are also qualitative defects of platelets, and abnormalities in both primary, release-independent, and secondary, release-dependent, aggregation have been noted [119, 146, 151, 231, 397]. In a quantitative study of various aspects of platelet function we have shown that although there is little evidence of an abnormal primary response to ADP, there is a consistent slight reduction in the primary reponse to adrenaline [397]. In addition, at least in some patients, there is a general reduction in platelet responses to all stimuli that partly or wholly depend on platelet granule secretion. Studies of accumulation storage and release of radiolabelled 5-hydroxytryptamine (5-HT) in the presence of specific inhibitors showed a reduced granule storage capacity in most patients, and this was most marked in those with a reduction in aggregation to several agents and with the most prolonged bleeding times [397]. This demonstration of a reduced granule storage pool is consistent with our impression that very dense bodies are rarely seen in HCL platelets: in our patient with the most reduced granule storage capacity, a detailed ultrastructural study of the platelets showed a marked reduction of very dense bodies. We therefore conclude that a granular storage pool defect is at least partly responsible for aggregation abnormalities in HCL, particularly as the platelet release reaction in response to thrombin appeared to be normal in these patients.

There is no direct evidence concerning the underlying mechanism or cause of the storage pool defect in HCL. The platelet dysfunction does not bear a simple relationship to thrombocytopenia, for platelet abnormalities have been observed in patients with a normal platelet count [151, 231, 397]. Moreover, although some improvement of platelet aggregation has been observed after splenectomy [119, 397], splenomegaly cannot be the general underlying cause, since some of our splenectomized patients showed abnormal platelet storage of 5-HT [397]. For the same reason, splenic sequestration of platelets seems an unlikely general cause of the platelet defect: indeed, in the one patient we have studied, platelet survival was normal [397].

Most HCL patients run a chronic course uncomplicated by any of the factors known to predispose to a platelet storage pool defect acquired in the circulation [287, 394]. Direct involvement of the megakaryocytic series in the underlying cell proliferation of HCL seems unlikely. The platelet abnormalities of HCL, like those of other cell types in the disease, are therefore probably attributable to disturbed marrow architecture and vasculature following fibrosis and infiltration by HCs, with the additional possibility that HCs produce humoral factors that specifically inhibit different cell series in the marrow.

6.4 Lymphocytes

6.4.1 T Cells

It is becoming increasingly recognized that T cells may be abnormal in a variety of haematological malignancies, and this is true in HCL.

Before discussing the abnormalities of T cells in HCL, some discussion of normal human T-cell subpopulations is necessary, since the nature, function, and interaction of T-cell subsets are complex and imperfectly understood.

The recognition of human T-cell heterogeneity has been limited by the lack of alloantisera, so that useful identification and functional analysis of human T-cell subsets have only recently become possible. MORETTA et al. [263, 265] were able to classify E rosette-forming T cells in normal human peripheral blood into those expressing a receptor for IgM after culture (Tμ), those with a receptor for IgG (Tγ), and those expressing neither receptor (To). Functional analysis of these subpopulations [266] revealed that Tμ cells acted as helper cells in the PWM-induced differentiation of B cells into plasma cells. Tμ cells may be the counterpart of the T_{H1} cells lysed by an absorbed heteroantiserum to peripheral T lymphocytes [82]. Tγ cells, on the other hand, after reaction with IgG immune complexes, acted as suppressor cells in B-cell differentiation [266]. The Tμ cells appeared to be a morphologically homogeneous population of small lymphocytes with a high nuclear : cytoplasmic ratio [24, 161], which gave a characteristic localized dot pattern of staining with NSE [161] and acid phosphatase [24]. Tγ cells were larger lymphocytes with a lower nuclear : cytoplasmic ratio, which were either negative or gave a scattered granular pattern with esterase and acid phosphatase cytochemistry [24, 161]. The transformation of Tμ and Tγ cells in response to PHA also differed [265], Tμ cells responding normally at a high concentration of PHA, while Tγ cells did not transform. However, over a range of PHA dilutions, a mixture of Tμ and Tγ cells gave a greater proliferative response than isolated Tμ cells.

This simple classification has recently been complicated by a number of observations.

1) *Tγ cells treated with IgG immune complexes* rapidly lose the γFc receptor and become To cells [262, 295]. After prolonged culture in medium containing foetal calf serum, a small proportion of these cells re-express the γFc receptor, but the majority acquire μFc receptors and become apparent Tμ cells [295].

2) *When purified T cells are reacted with IgG immune complexes*, the majority of Tμ cells lose the characteristic dot-staining pattern observed with esterase and acid phosphatase cytochemistry [24]. Whether this is the result of direct interaction between IgG and Tμ cells or is attributable to factors released by Tγ cells on exposure to IgG is not yet clear.

3) *When T-cell subpopulations are purified* by positive enrichment of Tμ or Tγ by rosette formation with the relevant IgM or IgG antibody-sensitized erythrocytes (EAM or EAG respectively), almost pure subpopulations can be obtained [266, 295]. Similarly, with negative enrichment, the removal of Tγ cells by EAG-rosette formation results in a purified population of Tμ cells [266, 295]. However, the removal of Tμ cells by EAM-rosette formation results in an almost pure population of To cells, with no apparent enrichment of Tγ cells [265, 295]. The explanation of this observation is unknown, but it again indicates modulation of T-cell subsets after exposure to immune complexes.

4) *If purified T "helper" cells are cultured* in concanavalin A before being tested in the PWM induced B-cell differentiation system they act as suppressor cells [172].

5) *Cell-mediated killing by T cells in man* is very complex and probably involves both Tμ and Tγ cells and other as yet undefined T-cell subsets [e.g., 132, 371]. In addition, interactions of different T-cell types are important in specific cell-mediated killing [82].

6) *The normal range for Tμ, Tγ, and To cells* in peripheral blood varies considerably for different individuals and different laboratories. In purified T-cell preparations the percentage of cells expressing μFc receptors after culture (Tμ) has ranged from 36%–91%, with a variety of mean values from different laboratories, e.g., 52% [263], 35% [251], 79% [295], 56% [24]. Reported percentages of Tγ cells have varied from 5%–38%, with means given as 7%–10% [263, 266], 22% [295], and 23% [24]. To cells have been established as about 20% [24, 266] or 0% [295] of normal peripheral T cells.

These uncertainties about normal human T-lymphocyte subsets, their different types, numbers, and interactions, make it difficult to define possible abnormalities in haematological malignancy. However, some definite abnormalities have now been demonstrated. For example in CLL, Tμ cells are relatively deficient [86] and there is a corresponding decrease in the helper capacity of isolated T cells [86, 130]. But in most cases the functional T-cell defect is manifest only in the lack of help given normal allogeneic B cells to differentiate and secrete specific antibody following exposure to antigen [86]; the helper activity by T cells in the mitogen-induced differentiation of allogeneic B cells is normal in most cases [86, 130]. Thus the data provided by Fu et al. [86, 130] could be interpreted as indicating a clonal expansion of functionally normal T cells already committed to recognizing the same antigen as the idiotypic determinants of the monoclonal SIg on the B CLL cells. Also in CLL, T-lymphocyte colony formation is defective in a mitogen-stimulated double-layer culture technique [95, 126].

There are also abnormalities of the T-cell populations in HCL. Some T-cell deficiencies are evident during the "stable phase" of the disease when HCs predominate in the peripheral blood, and others become evident during the T-cell phase (see Sect. 2.6.2).

During the stable phase there appears to be a deficiency of Tμ cells, whether these are demonstrated by EAM-rosette formation or by esterase cytochemistry (Table 6.1). This deficiency of Tμ cells may account for the reduced PHA-induced transformation shown by

Table 6.1. Subpopulation analysis of cultured T cells[a] in HCL

Patient	Phase of the disease[b]	% Rosette formation[c]				Tμ esterase staining %[e]
		E	Tμ	Tγ	To[d]	
AB	Stable	78	5	40	> 30	32
DC	T-cell	92	0	22	> 70	21
HD	T-cell	100	15	5	80	22
NW	T-cell	87	12	16	> 50	16
Normal[f]		90 ± 6	56 ± 12	23 ± 12	≃ 20	62 ± 7

[a] T cells negatively enriched by removal of plastic-adherent monocytes and SIg-positive cells were cultured for 20 h in TC199 + 10% foetal calf serum
[b] See Sect. 2.6.2
[c] Cells rosetted with sheep erythrocytes (E) or with ox erythrocytes coated with rabbit anti-ox IgM (detecting Tμ) or IgG (detecting Tγ)
[d] Estimate of T cells lacking both μFc and γFc receptors
[e] Tμ cells identified by distinctive localized dot pattern of reactivity [24, 161]
[f] Mean and standard deviation of six normal individuals tested with the same reagents

purified T cells from cases of HCL [96, 101, 375], especially since this impaired response is not corrected by the addition of normal monocytes and is therefore not attributable to the monocytopenia of the disease [375].

As is shown in Table 6.1, the decrease in Tμ cells is accompanied by a reciprocal increase of To cells. The significance of this finding is not clear, but since immune complexes may be a feature of the disease (see Sect. 2.7.2 and 5.2.6), it may conceivably be due to constant in vivo conversion of Tγ to To cells by IgG complexes [262, 295].

Our cytochemical studies with NSE and acid phosphatase stains provide further evidence that the T cells in HCL are abnormal. Thus, these stains produce very similar dot activity in most normal T cells [24]; but in HCL frequently many more small lymphocytes give the dot pattern with NSE than with acid phosphatase staining and, occasionally, the reverse is the case. We can give no explanation for this abnormality in the T cells of HCL, but it is interesting to note that lack of concordance in T-acid phosphatase and esterase staining is observed in a proportion of T-cell lymphomas [230]. On the other hand, and in contrast to the T cells of CLL, the peripheral T cells of HCL during the stable phase appear to provide normal helper activity in the antigen-induced differentiation of allogeneic B cells [86], and can form normal numbers of T-cell colonies in in vitro experiments [126]. Splenic T cells in the disease also appear to proliferate normally in mixed lymphocyte culture reactions [96].

Some of the abnormalities of the T cells in HCL observed during the T-cell phase have been discussed in Sect. 2.6.2. Like the T cells during the stable phase, the T-cell population is relatively deficient in Tμ cells (Table 6.1), and there is frequently a lack of agreement in numbers of cells giving the dot pattern of staining activity with NSE and acid phosphatase. During this phase the T cells of some cases appear to transform normally to PHA [69, 76] but are defective in in vitro colony formation [126]. The distinctive morphology of many of these cells (Fig. 2.6) and the intracytoplasmic IgD to be found in the cells of most cases [48, 76] have already been discussed in Sect. 2.6.2.

All these points make it clear that HCL may be characterized by abnormalities in T-cell subpopulations. The study of hybrid cases (Sect. 5.6) and of patients in the T-cell phase of the disease (Sect. 2.6.2) suggest that T cells may, at least sometimes, be directly involved in the neoplastic proliferation.

6.4.2 B Cells

In HCL, as in other B-cell malignancies [55, 57, 136, 137, 255, 304], the proliferative monoclonal cells of the disease almost completely replace the normal B-cell component [57].

Although many cases of HCL have less than 50% morphologically identifiable HCs [28, 149, 373], there is evidence that in a substantial proportion of cases many more circulating lymphoid cells are involved in the leukaemic process. For example, we have demonstrated R-L complexes in cells that would otherwise be regarded as normal lymphocytes (Fig. 6.2) [57]. Again, TRAP and esterase staining often reveal many more pathological cells than are apparent in simple Romanowsky preparations (see Chap. 4). Immunofluorescence studies with an anti-Ia-like serum and with a specific anti-HC serum (which did not stain normal T or B cells) indicate that virtually all non-T cells, including many lymphoid cells not readily identifiable morphologically as HCs, stain with both antisera (Table 5.2). Finally, studies of surface immunoglobulin further substantiate this concept, since the percentage of cells bearing the exlusive light-chain type is often much higher than the percentage of morphologically unequivocal HCs [57].

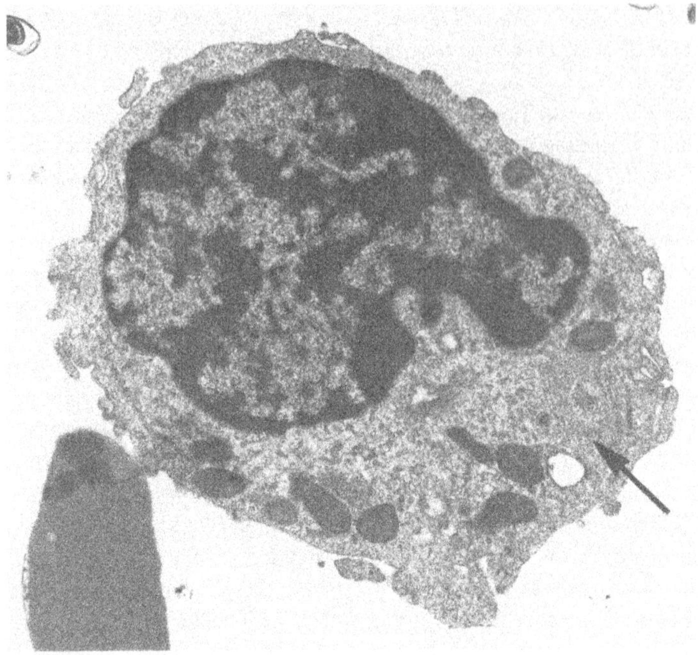

Fig. 6.2. R-L complex in a lymphocyte. This cell is not readily distinguishable from a normal lymphocyte – there are no typical surface projections and the nucleus contains moderately heavy peripheral chromatin condensation. However, the presence of a R-L complex (sectioned largely transversely) indicates that the cell is involved in the leukaemic proliferation (× 11,000)

As a corollary to this concept, it seems that circulating normal B lymphocytes are profoundly depressed in HCL. The number of cells bearing SIg light chains of the type not involved in the clonal proliferation is strikingly low, even when highly sensitive methods are employed [58, 315]. With immunofluorescent methods it has frequently been recorded, but not commented upon, that there are virtually no cells bearing the nonpredominant light-chain type [2, 33, 102, 129, 166, 191, 232]. Similarly, since normal B lymphocytes have receptors for C3b [321] and form rosettes with yeast particles coated with C3b [50, 256], the virtual absence of such rosettes in HCL [50] also indicates an absence of normal B lymphocytes in the disease. A deficiency of cells of the normal B-cell series, which is a feature of several B-cell malignancies, may be due to negative feedback mechanisms [344]. This may be true of HCL, but the absence of immuneparesis and the polyclonal nature of the tissue plasma cells in the disease (see Chap. 3) both suggest that specific blocking of B-cell maturation does not occur.

7 Diagnosis

7.1 Differential Diagnosis

Appreciation of the distinctive clinicopathological picture of HCL should enable the correct diagnosis to be readily made in the great majority of cases. Careful examination of the blood film in an adult with splenomegaly but without substantial lymphadenopathy will almost invariably reveal the presence of pathognomonic HCs if HCL is the diagnosis. When a leucopenia is present there is an added incentive to be particularly thorough in this search, and if the patient is very leucopenic it may be necessary to examine a buffy-coat preparation. Failure to make the presumptive diagnosis at this stage is most likely to be due to lack of familiarity with the entity and its diagnostic HC. In our experience, HCs are never completely absent from the peripheral blood at presentation, and in those patients with a leucocytosis HCs are always frequent. The paucity of neutrophils and monocytes so characteristic of the disease forms part of the initial diagnostic impression. The HCs themselves are often more readily identified away from the tail of the film.

Subsequent investigations are either largely confirmatory or serve to exclude the occasional case of non-Hodgkin's lymphoma that may present a similar picture. Acid-phosphatase staining should reveal strong scattered granular activity not inhibited by tartrate (TRAP) in the putative HCs. Weak TRAP activity is not diagnostic, since it may be observed in a variety of other lymphoid cells; even strong activity may very occasionally be misleading, since it has been reported in a variety of other cell types [63, 204, 225, 241, 267, 271, 279, 381, 388]. Cases of HCL without strong TRAP activity have been reported [40, 204, 340], but with the technique based on naphthyl ASBI phosphate and fast garnet GBC (Sect. 4.2.1), we have found clear positivity in all cases.

Additional observations that may be useful at this stage are a high LAP score (in typical HCL the LAP score is > 150 [171]) and a raised MCV on the Coulter S.

Electron microscopy readily confirms the presence of HCs and may reveal distinctive R-L complexes (Sect. 4.3.1).

A bone marrow aspirate should be attempted. This will frequently be unsuccessful, but a dry tap is of diagnostic significance. Hairy cells may appear less hairy in bone-marrow smears, but at least some of the mononuclear cells will be typical HCs, and others can be identified as such by their characteristic nucleus and distinctive slate-blue cytoplasm. Whether or not aspiration is successful, a trephine biopsy should be performed. The demonstration of an increase in reticulin, together with a mononuclear infiltrate and depression of other marrow elements, is frequently the final diagnostic criterion (Sect. 3.1). If the patient undergoes splenectomy, the diagnosis should always be confirmed retrospectively by the demonstration of diffuse involvement of the red pulp both macroscopically and microscopically (Sect. 3.2).

The list of conditions with which HCL has been confused is long and includes a variety of non-Hodgkin's lymphomas, chronic lymphocytic leukaemia, Waldenström's macroglobulinaemia, myelofibrosis, a variety of monocytic and histiocytic proliferations, Sézary's syndrome, acute undifferentiated and lymphoblastic leukaemia, and aplastic anaemia [16, 28, 40, 61, 70, 121, 149, 202, 239, 298, 337, 370, 373, 390]. Nevertheless, if the criteria outlined above are fulfilled, there will rarely be diagnostic confusion. Perhaps the only sources of real diagnostic difficulty are certain non-Hodgkin's lymphomas and the entity described in the next section. For example, we have observed occasional patients, who proved to have non-Hodgkin's lymphoma, who had presented with substantial splenomegaly, inconspicuous or absent lymphadenopathy, peripheral pancytopenia (including neutropenia and monocytopenia), and prominent mononuclear cells in the peripheral blood and bone marrow, some of which appeared to be HCs. However, many of the supposed HCs were slightly different from typical HCs, the surface hairs being too thick and short and the nuclear chromatin slightly too condensed. They frequently contained TRAP, but this activity was not strong. The LAP score was not elevated, and electron microscopy confirmed the cytological differences from typical HCs and failed to reveal R-L complexes. KATAYAMA's group [210, 279] have described cases of lymphoma that could lead to similar difficulty, and have emphasized the importance of histopathology of bone marrow, spleen, and lymph node in distinguishing them from HCL.

Finally, we have observed that certain immunological tests (Sect. 5.5) which are largely investigative may occasionally be of diagnostic assistance in differentiating HCL from non-Hodgkin's lymphoma presenting a similar clinical and haematological picture. For example, the absence of receptors for the Fc of IgM and IgG, the presence of C3 receptors, and the demonstration of SIgM and SIgD only would all argue against the diagnosis of HCL.

7.2 A New Distinct Entity

We have seen two patients (a woman aged 64 and a man aged 72 years) with a disease closely resembling HCL in a number of respects, but with certain differences perhaps justifying its recognition as a distinct entity [75].

In both patients the disease was chronic and there were no significant constitutional symptoms. Both patients had massive splenomegaly (> 20 cm below costal margin) but no hepatomegaly or lymphadenopathy. Numerous mononuclear cells with a strikingly hairy appearance (in ROMANOWSKY-stained smears and in phase-contrast preparations) (Figs. 7.1 and 7.2) and strong TRAP activity were present in the peripheral blood. The bone marrow

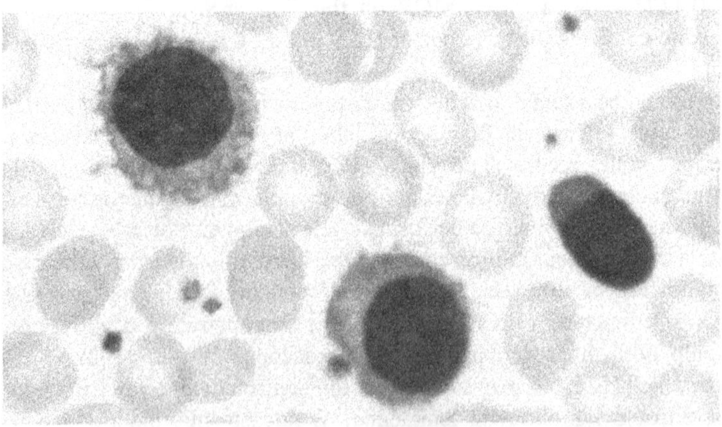

Fig. 7.1. "Hairy cells" of a possible new distinct entity (ROMANOWSKY preparation). One of the cells closely resembles a typical HC, but the other cell, although distinctly hairy, has a nucleus with heavily condensed chromatin

was diffusely infiltrated by large numbers of similar cells, and in the one patient who has been splenectomized these cells totally replaced the normal splenic architecture and diffusely infiltrated the red pulp. Repeated immunological studies of the "hairy cells" from both patients showed that these were phagocytic for latex particles and had a surface-marker phenotype typical of HCL [$E^{-}SIg^{+}(1\kappa,1\lambda)\gamma Fc^{+}\mu Fc^{+}C3^{-}Mo^{-}$; see Sect. 5.5].
However, the disease differed from typical HCL in a number of important respects. Both patients had a marked leucocytosis at presentation ($> 50 \times 10^9$/litre). Both ROMANOWSKY (Figs. 7.1 and 7.3) and ultrastructural study (Fig. 7.4) showed that the "hairy cells" were atyp-

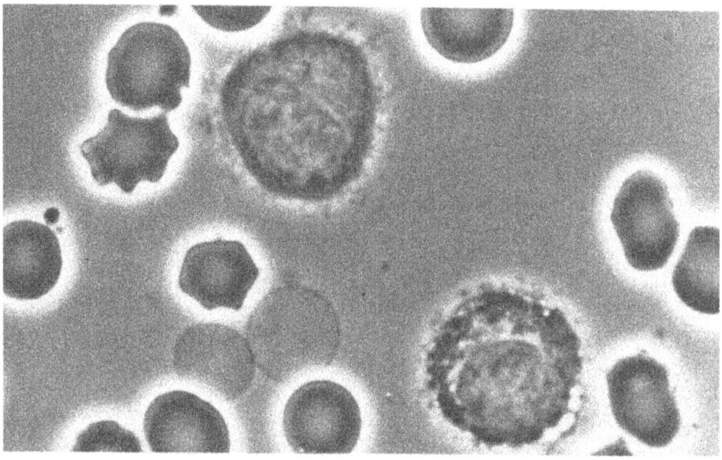

Fig. 7.2. "Hairy cells" of a possible new distinct entity (phase-contrast preparation). These cells are indistinguishable from those of typical HCL

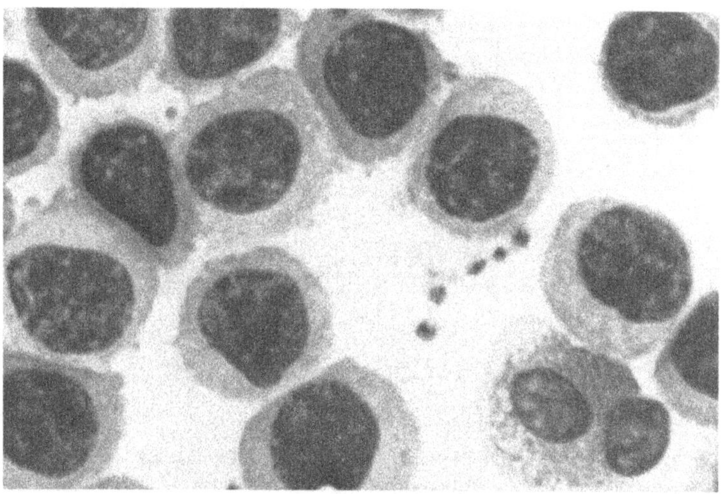

Fig. 7.3. "Hairy cells" of a possible new distinct entity (ROMANOWSKY preparation). The cells are clearly atypical in a number of respects. The nuclei are more rounded and regular than those of typical HCs and contain more heterochromatin. Although some fine surface hairs are seen, many are coarser than those characteristic of HCs. This picture was taken in the tail of the film where even typical HCs appear somewhat less hairy

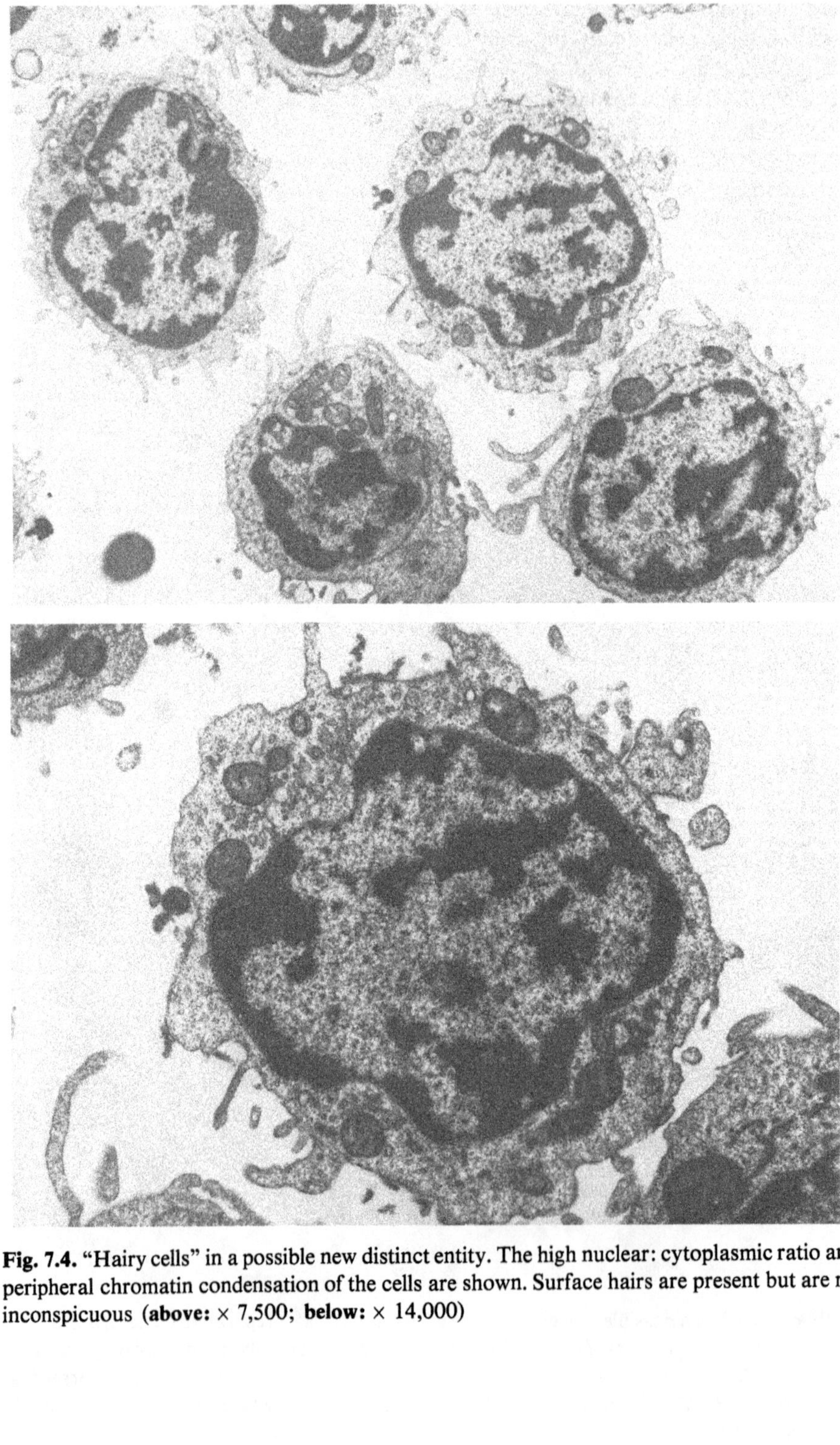

Fig. 7.4. "Hairy cells" in a possible new distinct entity. The high nuclear: cytoplasmic ratio and heavy peripheral chromatin condensation of the cells are shown. Surface hairs are present but are relatively inconspicuous (**above:** × 7,500; **below:** × 14,000)

ical in possessing moderately heavy heterochromatin and a high nuclear : cytoplasmic ratio. The nucleolus was frequently more prominent than in typical HCs and the surface projections were not as conspicuous on TEM (Fig. 7.4). Ribosome-lamella complexes were not observed, although fibrillary inclusions (Sect. 4.3.1) were conspicuous in one of the patients. The marrow proved easy to aspirate, and bone biopsy showed that reticulin was not markedly increased. Monocytopenia and neutropenia were not prominent features of the blood film, and marrow myelopoiesis was not as profoundly depressed as in typical HCL. Some of the monocytes from one of the cases appeared abnormal (Fig. 7.5). The LAP score was not elevated in either patient and the strong TRAP activity was somewhat atypical in frequently being concentrated at one pole of the cell. The high nuclear : cytoplasmic ratio and heavy chromatin condensation of the infiltrating mononuclear cells were evident in splenic sections from one patient. In one of the cases, the "hairy cells"were highly phagocytic for IgG-opsonized erythrocytes (Fig. 7.6) [51]; in the other case the pathological cells were slightly more phagocytic for these particles than are typical HCs. One patient had a small paraprotein peak (IgGk) without immuneparesis and the other had immuneparesis without a paraprotein peak.

These two cases are clearly different from the type of non-Hodgkin's lymphoma described by NEIMAN et al. [279] and KATAYAMA [201], in which there are a few circulating "hairy cells" and which can thus be confused with HCL. They are also distinct from both prolymphocytic (PLL) and chronic lymphocytic leukaemia (CLL), which are the two main differential diagnoses. In particular, the constitutional symptoms of PLL were lacking and the cells, in addition to being strikingly hairy, did not possess the very large prominent nucleoli characteristic of prolymphocytes [134]. The absence of lymphadenopathy, the strong TRAP activity present in many of the abnormal cells, the marked phagocytic ability of the cells, the conspicuous fibrillary inclusions, and the absence of Mo-rosette formation were further features distinguishing the two cases from CLL.

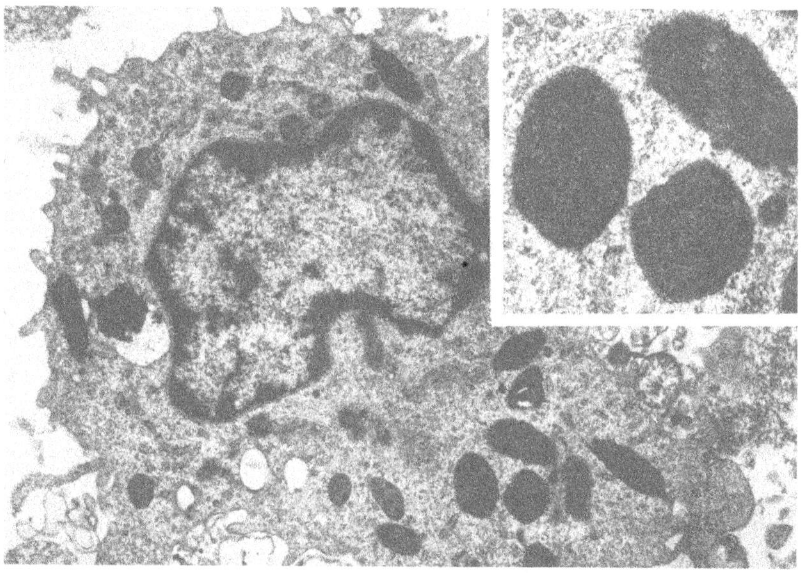

Fig. 7.5. Abnormal monocyte in the possible new distinct entity. Most of the granules are abnormally large and, as is clearly shown in the *inset*, display a distinct substructure (× 11,000; *inset* × 29,500)

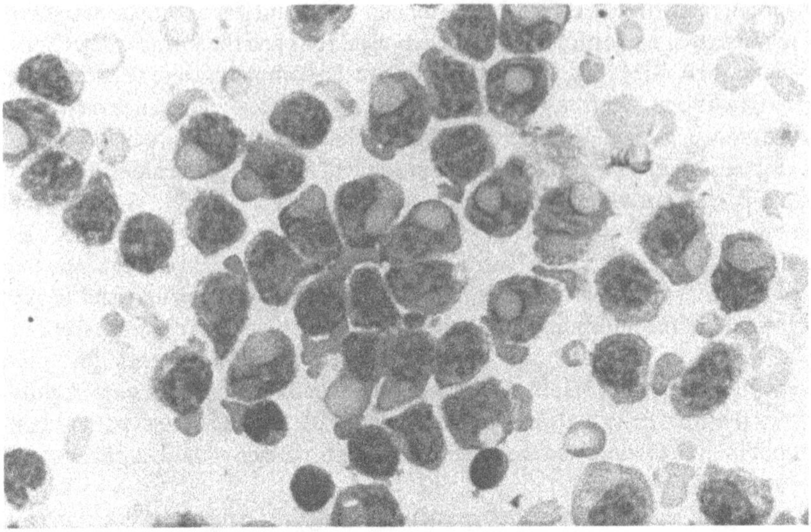

Fig. 7.6. Phagocytosis of IgG-opsonized erythrocytes. The "hairy cells" are strongly phagocytic for these particles. Nonopsonized erythrocytes were not phagocytosed

Both our patients have continued to run a chronic and relatively asymptomatic course and are alive and well some 4 and 2 years after presentation. Chlorambucil caused some reduction in the leucocyte count, and splenectomy in one case and splenic irradiation in the other have been beneficial in removing splenic discomfort.

8 Conclusions and Future Trends

The last 10 years have seen an increasingly active interest in HCL. This interest has been wide-ranging, and the clinical, haematological, cytological, pathological, and immunological characteristics of the disease are now well established; all these have confirmed that HCL is a specific disease entity.

Hairy-cell leukemia can almost always be correctly diagnosed with relatively few simple investigations. Certain non-Hodgkin's lymphomas with isolated splenomegaly, peripheral pancytopenia, and mononuclear cells bearing some resemblance to HCs may occasionally present diagnostic difficulties, but such cases can usually be distinguished from HCL by careful attention to cytological, cytochemical, and histological detail. Future studies may further characterize a related, but distinct, entity with isolated splenomegaly and a florid leukaemia involving HCs distinguishable from those of HCL. The precise relationship of these disorders to typical HCL is not yet established.

Accurate diagnosis of HCL has important prognostic and therapeutic implications, for if erythropoiesis is not compromised the prognosis is usually good and vigorous chemotherapy is contraindicated during most of the course of the disease. Patients are often relatively young and, especially if they survive the first 2 years of illness, can be expected to live for prolonged periods. The most important prognostic factor is probably the degree of marrow impairment present.

Elective splenectomy should be recommended in patients with substantial splenomegaly, especially if the splenic red-cell volume is clearly increased. In other patients and in those unfit for operation steroids may be useful. Other forms of chemotherapy should be reserved for patients with severely compromised marrow function who have either failed to respond to splenectomy or relapsed following initial improvement after this procedure. In general, only if such patients have shown no substantial improvement after gentle chemotherapy, including steroids alone, should vigorous cytotoxic regimes be employed. At this stage of the illness, their management resembles that of patients with acute myeloid leukaemia (AML), and, with intensive supportive care, a few patients will achieve remission. Dramatic therapeutic advances for patients with profound marrow impairment, as in AML, will probably require the development of new drugs or new therapeutic concepts.

Chemotherapeutic restraint is further encouraged by the fact that marked fluctuations may be observed in the course of the disease, particularly after splenectomy. Sometimes patients may show apparently spontaneous improvement lasting many months. It has been demonstrated that these fluctuations are accompanied by a disappearance of circulating HCs and by immunological changes, including complex alterations in the peripheral T-cell populations. Since the disease is subjected to relatively little therapeutic intervention, HCL is particularly suitable for the recognition and study of fluctuations in its natural history. It is possible, however, that spontaneous alterations associated with T-cell population abnormalities will prove to be a general feature of chronic lymphoproliferative disorders.

Despite intensive investigations with a variety of techniques, the origins of the HC are still elusive. The HC has a number of characteristics, all of which are almost peculiar to this cell and which, taken together, define the HC and distinguish it from other pathological cells and from known normal haemic cell types.

It is possible that the unique combination of characteristics defining the HC arises as a result of malignancy-induced alterations of a well-recognized haemic cell type, but this has not proved to be true in those haematological malignancies in which the normal counterpart is known. It is more likely that the HC arises from a still unidentified mononuclear cell population. If this is so, it seems fallacious to attempt to place HCs within a particular cell lineage on the basis of one or other of the characteristics it shares with cells of that line, while disregarding equally prominent distinguishing features. Definitive classification of a cell type depends on knowledge of its functional capabilities; little is known about the physiological capacity of HCs. Hairy cells share marker characteristics with monocytes, B lymphocytes, T lymphocytes and third-population cells, so that classification on marker criteria alone, without reference to function, depends upon the emphasis given to any particular marker. For example, the presence of surface immunoglobulin on HCs has led to HCL being widely regarded as a B-cell disorder. However, HCs lack some of the markers of B cells and possess other features not normally associated with these cells; furthermore the tissue distribution of HCs is quite unlike that of known B-cell subsets. In addition, HCs have not been shown to be capable of differentiating into Ig-secreting plasma cells – an essential characteristic of B cells.

The evidence favouring a monocytic lineage, including strong glass adherence, phagocytic ability, and the specific infiltration of the splenic red pulp, is weakened by the fact that HCs manufacture Ig and lack many of the characteristics of monocytes, particularly the ability to differentiate into functional macrophages.

The HC possesses certain features in common with some T cells (particularly $T\gamma$ cells). Thus, T-cell cases of HCL are not rare, and weak E-rosette formation by HCs is frequently observed. Isoenzyme 5 (TRAP) acid-phosphatase activity, and the ability to support replication of Herpes simplex virus are also features common to HCs and some T lymphoblasts. Clearly, however, HCs have many characteristics not shared by T cells, and have not been shown to possess the helper- or suppressor-cell capacity of T-cell subpopulations.

Again, the HC possesses features of the imperfectly understood cells of the third-population, or null-cell group. At least some of the cells in this group bear strong γFc receptors, some can form weak E rosettes, and some Ia-positive cells from this group can synthesize Ig. Although HCs cannot effect antibody-dependent, cell-mediated cytotoxicity (a function of K cells present in this third-population cell group), the function of many third-population cells is not known; the normal counterpart of the HC may be present within this ill-understood heterogeneous minority population.

Whatever the precise nature of HCs, the extensive knowledge of their markers accumulated in recent years will eventually prove of wider value, not only in identifying the normal counterpart of the HC itself but also in helping to clarify normal human lymphocyte heterogeneity. Many of the perplexing features of HCL will be clarified with further advances in the understanding of the structure and function of the lymphoreticular system. For example, the reason why HCs take on the distribution of reticuloendothelial cells may become more readily understood as the factors determining the distribution and migration of haemic cells become better defined. Finally, elucidation of the function of HCs and their possible effects on other cell types may eventually explain such features as the selective monocytopenia and neutropenia so characteristic of HCL.

9 References

1 Advani SH, Talwalker GV, Nadkarni JS, Nadkarni JJ, Sirsat SM, Srinivasan U (1976) Hairy cell leukaemia. A case report and review of literature. Indian J Cancer 13:283–287

2 Aisenberg AC, Bloch KJ, Long JC (1973) Cell-surface immunoglobulins in chronic lymphocytic leukemia and allied disorders. Am J Med 55:184–191

3 Alexander E, Sanders S (1978) Fc receptor bearing 'hairy cells' of leukaemic reticuloendotheliosis bind soluble antigen-antibody complexes and adhere to immobilized complexes, but fail to mediate antibody dependent cellular cytotoxicity. Scand J Immunol 8:477–488

4 Alonso CM, Bernabe RR, Moreno E, de Espada FD (1978) Depletion of monocytes from human peripheral blood leucocytes by passage through Sephadex G-10 columns. J Immunol Methods 22:361–368

5 Alptuna E, Anteunis A, Krulik M, Astesano A, Robineaux R, Debray J (1978) Hairy cell leukemia: a clinical, immunological and ultrastructural study. New data for the origin of the hairy cell. Virchows Archiv [Cell Pathol] 28:135–149

6 Amlot PL, Adinolfi M (1979) Serum β2 microglobulin and its prognostic value in lymphomas. Eur J Cancer 15:791–796

7 Anday GJ, Goodman JR, Tishkoff GH (1973) An unusual cytoplasmic ribosomal structure in pathological lymphocytes. Blood 41:439–449

8 Anderson RE, Walford RL (1963) Fibroblastic type of leukemic reticuloendotheliosis. Cancer 16:993–997

9 Andersson LC (1979) Personal communication

10 Andersson LC, Gahmberg CG (1978) Surface glycoproteins of human white blood cells. Analysis by surface labelling. Blood 52:57–67

11 Andersson LC, Gahmberg CG, Siimes MA, Teerenhovi L , Vuopio P (1979) Cell surface glycoprotein analysis: a diagnostic tool in human leukemias. Int J Cancer 23:306–311

12 Annals of the New York Academy of Sciences (1978) Fibroblast surface protein. 312

13 Banerjee D, Hamdy H, Bormanis J, Walker T, Richter M (1978) Leukemic reticuloendotheliosis: polyclonal surface immunoglobulin on 'hairy' cells. Cancer 41:1804–1810

14 Barker CR, Burns GF, Cawley JC, Hayhoe FGJ (1976) IgM receptors on the surface of hairy cells of leukaemic reticuloendotheliosis. Lancet 1:1303

15 Barrett I (to be published) Steroid receptors of the pathological cells in hairy-cell and chronic lymphocytic leukaemia

16 Bauters F, Latte J, Jouet JP, Goudemand J, Goudemand M (1979) La leucémie à tricholeucocytes: étude clinique, hématologique et évolutive. Lille Med 22:306–315

17 Beachey EH, Hashimota K, Burkett LL (1969) Histiocytic leukemia: ultrastructure and phagocytic capacity of hairy cells. Clin Res 17:530

18 Belding HW, Daland GA, Parker F (1955) Histiocytic and monocytic leukemia. A clinical, haematological, and pathological differentiation. Cancer 8:237–252

19 Belpomme D, Borella L, Braylan R, Greaves M, Herberman R, Hitzig W, Kersey J, Petrov R, Ritts R, Seligmann M, Sobin L, Thierfelder S, Torrigiani G (1978) Immunological diagnosis of leukaemia and lymphoma: a World Health Organization/International Union of Immunological Societies technical report. Br J Haematol 38:85–98

20 Bentwich Z, Douglas SD, Siegal FP, Kunkel HG (1973) Human lymphocyte-sheep erythrocyte rosette formation: some characteristics of the interaction. Clin Immunol Immunopathol 1:511–522

21 Berg B, Brandt L (1970) The cytology, distribution and function of the neoplastic cells in leukaemic reticuloendotheliosis. Scand J Haematol 7:428–434

22 Bertoglio J, Peaud PY, Byron PA, Treille D, Felman P, Doré JF (1976) Prognostic value of mouse red cell rosette formation in chronic lymphocytic leukaemia. Biomedicine [Express] 25:277–278

23 Besa EC, Dale DC, Wolff SM, Gardner FH (1975) Etiocholanolone and prednisolone therapy in patients with severe bone marrow failure. Proceedings of XVII Annual Meeting of the American Society of Haematology, Dallas, Texas

24 Bevan A, Burns GF, Grey L, Cawley JC (1980) Cytochemistry of human T-cell subpopulations. Scand J Immunol 11:223–233

25 Bodel PT, Nichols BA, Bainton DF (1978) Differences in peroxidase reactivity within the rough endoplasmic reticulum of blood monocytes after adherence. J Exp Med 145:264–274

26 Boiron M, Flandrin G, Ripault J, Lortholary P, Teillet F, Jacquillat C, Bernard J (1968) Histiolymphocytose médullaire et splénique d'apparence primitive. Nouv Rev Fr Hématol 8:179–200

27 Boldt DH, Speckart SF, MacDermott RP, Nash GS, Valeski JE (1977) Leukemic reticuloendotheliosis. "Hairy cell leukemia", functional and structural features of the abnormal cell in a patient with profound leukocytosis. Blood 49:745–757

28 Bouroncle BA (1979) Leukemic reticuloendotheliosis (hairy cell leukemia). Blood 53:412–436

29 Bouroncle BA, Wiseman BK, Doan CA (1958) Leukemic reticuloendotheliosis. Blood 13:609–630

30 Bouza E, Burgaleta C, Golde DW (1978) Infections in hairy-cell leukemia. Blood 51:851–859

31 Branda RF (1976) Leukemic Reticuloendotheliosis and 'Hairy Cells'. N Engl J Med 295:1015

32 Braunsteiner VH, Schmalzl F, Asamer H (1974) Zytologische Untersuchungen bei „hairy-cell"-Leukämien. Acta Med Austriaca 1:35–41

33 Braylan RC, Jaffe ES, Triche TJ, Nanba K, Fowlkes BJ, Metzger H, Frank MM, Dolan MS, Yee CL, Green I, Berard CW (1978) Structural and functional properties of the 'hairy' cells of leukemic reticuloendotheliosis. Cancer 41:210–227

34 Breton-Gorius J, Guichard J (1972) Ultrastructural localization of peroxidase activity in human platelets and megakaryocytes. Am J Pathol 66:277–293

35 Breton-Gorius J, Houssay D, Vilde JL, Dreyfus B (1975) Partial myeloperoxidase deficiency in a case of preleukaemia. II. Defects of degranulation and abnormal bactericidal activity of blood neutrophils. Br J Haematol 30:279–288

36 Brown G, Greaves MF, Lister TA, Rapson N, Papamichail M (1974) Expression of human T and B lymphocyte cell-surface markers on leukaemic cells. Lancet 2:753–755

37 Brunning RD, Parkin J (1975) Ribosome-lamella complexes in neoplastic haematopoietic cells. Am J Pathol 79:565–572

38 Bulger RE (1968) Granule-lamella complex in monkey renal proximal tubule cells. J Ultrastruct Res 24:150–156

39 Burke JS (1978) The value of the bone-marrow biopsy in the diagnosis of hairy cell leukemia. Am J Clin Pathol 70:876–884

40 Burke JS, Byrne GE Jr, Rappaport H (1974) Hairy cell leukemia (leukemic reticuloendotheliosis). I. A clinical pathologic study of 21 patients. Cancer 33:1399–1410

41 Burke JS, Mackay B, Rappaport H (1976) Hairy cell leukemia (leukemic reticuloendotheliosis). II. Ultrastructure of the spleen. Cancer 37:2267–2274

42 Burns CP, Hoak JC (1973) Freeze-etching, scanning and thin section electron microscopic studies of the "hairy" leucocytes in leukemic reticuloendotheliosis. J Natl Cancer Inst 51:743–750

43 Burns CP, Maca RD, Hoak JC (1973) Biochemical, morphological, and immunological observations of leukemic reticuloendotheliosis. Cancer Res 33:1615–1624

44 Burns GF, Cawley JC (1979) A re-examination of the alleged monocytic features of hairy-cell leukaemia. Scand J Haematol 22:386–396

45 Burns GF, Cawley JC (1979) The detection of membrane-associated complement components (C3b and C4b) on circulating human normal and leukaemic leucocytes and on cultured cells with monkey erythrocytes. Eur J Immunol 9:791–796

46 Burns GF, Cawley JC (1980) Spontaneous mouse erythrocyte-rosette formation: correlation with surface immunoglobulin phenotype in hairy-cell leukemia. Clin Exp Immunol 39:83–89

47 Burns GF, Cawley JC, Barker CR (1979) Characterization of the receptor for IgM present on human B lymphocytes. Immunology 36:569–577

48 Burns GF, Worman CP, Cawley JC (1980) Fluctuations in the T and B characteristics of two cases of T-cell hairy-cell leukaemia. Clin Exp Immunol 39:76–82

49 Burns GF, Barker CR, Cawley JC, Hayhoe FGJ (1977) The rate of membrane turnover by the hairy cells of leukemic reticuloendotheliosis: a kinetic study of a receptor for IgM. J Immunol 119:1279–1284

50 Burns GF, Cawley JC, Barker CR, Hayhoe FGJ (1977) Absence of a receptor for fixed C3 on the hairy cells of leukaemic reticuloendotheliosis. Clin Exp Immunol 29:442–446

51 Burns GF, Cawley JC, Barker CR, Goldstone AH, Hayhoe FGJ (1977) New evidence relating to the nature and origin of the hairy cell of leukaemic reticuloendotheliosis. Br J Haematol 36:71–84

52 Burns GF, Cawley JC, Worman CP, Barker CR, Hayhoe FGJ (1979) Distribution of a receptor for IgM (μFcR) on haemic cells. Am J Hematol 6:243–251

53 Burns GF, Flemans RJ, Barker CR, Cawley JC, Worman CP, Hayhoe FGJ (1976) Leukemic reticuloendotheliosis and 'hairy cells'. N Engl J Med 295:1015

54 Burns GF, Nash AA, Worman CP, Barker CR, Hayhoe FGJ, Cawley JC (1977) A human leukaemic cell expressing hybrid membrane phenotypes. Nature 268:243–245

55 Burns GF, Worman CP, Roberts BE, Raper CGL, Barker CR, Cawley JC (1979) Terminal B cell development as seen in different human myelomas and related disorders. Clin Exp Immunol 35:180–189

56 Burns GF, Cawley JC, Barker CR, Nash AA, Rees JKH, Worman CP, Hayhoe FGJ (1978) Kinetic studies of surface markers on the pathological cells of hairy cell leukaemia (HCL) and chronic lymphocytic leukaemia (CLL). In: Bentvelzen P, Hilgers J, Yohn DS (eds) Advances in comparative leukemia research. Elsevier/North Holland, Amsterdam

57 Burns GF, Cawley JC, Higgy KE, Barker CR, Edwards M, Rees JKH, Hayhoe FGJ (1978) Hairy-cell leukaemia: a B-cell neoplasm with a severe deficiency of circulating normal B lymphocytes. Leukemia Res 2:33–40

58 Burns GF, Cawley JC, Worman CP, Karpas A, Barker CR, Goldstone AH, Hayhoe FGJ (1978) Multiple heavy chain isotypes on the surface of the cells of hairy-cell leukemia. Blood 52:1132–1147

59 Carpentier NA, Lange GT, Fiere DM, Fournie GJ, Lambert P-H, Miescher PA (1977) Clinical relevance of circulating immune complexes in human leukemia. Association in acute leukemia of the presence of immune complexes with unfavourable prognosis. J Clin Invest 60:874–884

60 Case Records of the Massachusetts General Hospital. Case 21 (1977) N Engl J Med 296:1218–1225

61 Cassiere SG, Gregg R, Eichner ER (1977) Hairy cell leukaemia. Postgrad Med 61:231–233

62 Castro-Malaspina H, Najean Y, Flandrin G (1979) Erythrokinetic studies in hairy-cell leukaemia. Br J Haematol 42:189–197

63 Catovsky D (1977) Hairy-cell leukaemia and prolymphocytic leukaemia. Clin Haematol 6:245–268

64 Catovsky D, Galton DAG (1973) Lysozyme activity and nitroblue-tetrazolium reduction in leukaemic cells. J Clin Pathol 26:60–69

65 Catovsky D, Tripp E, Hoffbrand AV (1972) Response to phytohaemagglutinin and pokeweed mitogen in chronic lymphocytic leukaemia. Lancet 1:794–795

66 Catovsky D, Frisch B, Okos A, Noorden SV (1975) Scanning electron microscopy and the nature of the hairy cell. Lancet 1:462–463

67 Catovsky D, Cherchi M, Okos A, Hegde U, Galton DAG (1976) Mouse red-cell rosettes in B-lymphoproliferative disorders. Br J Haematol 33:173–177

68 Catovsky D, Papamichail M, Okos A, Miliani E, Holborow EJ (1975) Formation of mouse red cell rosettes by 'hairy' cells. Biomedicine 23:81–84

69 Catovsky D, Pettit JE, Galetto J, Okos A, Galton DAG (1974) The B-lymphocyte nature of the 'hairy' cell of leukaemic reticuloendotheliosis. Br J Haematol 26:29–37

70 Catovsky D, Pettit JE, Galton DAG, Spiers ASD, Harrison CV (1974) Leukaemic reticuloendotheliosis ('hairy' cell leukaemia): a distinct clinico-pathological entity. Br J Haematol 26:9–27

71 Catovsky D, Sperandio P, O'Brien M, Cherchi M, Galton DAG (1977) Phagocytic potential of leukaemic B-lymphocytes. Scand J Haematol 19:211–216

72 Cawley JC, Burns GF (1977) Studies relating to the nature and origin of the hairy cells of leukaemic reticuloendotheliosis. Q J Med 46:551

73 Cawley JC, Hayhoe FGJ (1973) Ultrastructure of haemic cells. Saunders, London

74 Cawley JC, Karpas A (1974) The ultrastructural demonstration of virus-like particles in human leukaemic cells. Eur J Cancer 10:559–562

75 Cawley JC, Burns GF, Hayhoe FGJ A distinct variant of hairy-cell leukaemia. Submitted for publication

76 Cawley JC, Burns GF, Worman CP, Roberts BE, Hayhoe FGJ (to be published 1980) Clinical and haematological fluctuations in hairy-cell leukaemia: a sequential surface-marker analysis. Blood

77 Cawley JC, Burns GF, Nash TA, Higgy KE, Child JA, Roberts BE (1978) Hairy-cell leukaemia with T-cell features. Blood 51:61–69

78 Cawley JC, Emmines J, Goldstone AH, Hamblin J, Hough D, Smith JL (1975) Distinctive cytoplasmic inclusions in chronic lymphocytic leukaemia. Eur J Cancer 11:91–92

79 Cawley JC, Burns GF, Worman CP, Bevan A, Hunt KM, Roberts BE, Hayhoe FGJ (1979) T-cell features in hairy-cell leukaemia. Br J Haematol 43:679–682

80 Cawley JC, Burns GF, Bevan A, Worman CP, Smith JL, Gray L, Barker CR, Hayhoe FGJ (1979) Typical hairy-cell leukaemia with IgGk paraproteinaemia. Br J Haematol 43:215–221

81 Charron D, Barrett AJ, Faille A, Alby N, Schmitt T, Degos L (1977) Lithium in acute myeloid leukaemia. Lancet 1:1307

82 Chess L, Schlossman SF (1977) Human lymphocyte subpopulations. Adv Immunol 25:213–241

83 Chess L, Levine H, MacDermott RP, Schlossman SF (1975) Immunologic functions of isolated human lymphocyte subpopulations. VI. Further characterization of the surface Ig negative, E rosette negative (null cell) subset. J Immunol 115:1483–1487

84 Child JA, Cawley JC, Martin S, Ghoneim ATM (1979) Microbicidal function of the neutrophils in hairy-cell leukaemia. Acta Haematol (Basel) 62:191–198

85 Child JA, Martin S, Cawley JC, Ghoneim ATM (1978) Defective microbicidal function of neutrophils in haematological malignancies and lymphomas: correction by levamisole in vitro. Biomedicine 29:159–161

86 Chiorazzi N, Fu SM, Montazeri G, Kunkel HG, Rail K, Gee T (1979) T cell helper defect in patients with chronic lymphocytic leukemia. J Immunol 122:1087–1090

87 Cicco de D, Greaves MF, Engh van den G, Warner NL (1978) Expression of cholera toxin binding sites on normal and malignant haemopoietic cells. In: Bentvelzen P, Hilgers J, Yohn DS (eds) Advances in comparative leukemia research. Elsevier/North Holland, Amsterdam

88 Cohen HJ, George ER, Kremer WB (1979) Hairy cell leukaemia: cellular characteristics including surface immunoglobulin dynamics and biosynthesis. Blood 53:764–775

89 Cohen HJ, Shimm D, Paris SA, Buckley CE, Kremer WB (1979) Hairy cell leukaemia-associated familial lymphoproliferative disorder. Ann Intern Med 90:174–179

90 Cooper MD, Seligmann M (1977) B and T lymphocytes in immunodeficiency and lymphoproliferative diseases. In: Loor F, Roelants GE (eds) B and T cells in immune recognition. Wiley, London

91 Cooper MD, Kearney JF, Lawton AR, Abney ER, Parkhouse RME, Preud'homme JL, Seligmann M (1976) Generation of immunoglobulin class diversity in B cells: a discussion with emphasis on IgD development. Ann Immunol (Paris) 127C:573–581

92 Daems W Th, Wisse E, Brederro P, Emeis JJ (1975) Peroxidatic activity in monocytes and macrophages. In: Van Furth R (ed) Mononuclear phagocytes in immunity, infection and pathology. Blackwell, Oxford

93 Daniel MT, Flandrin G (1974) Fine structure of abnormal cells in hairy cell leukemia, with special reference to their in vitro phagocytic capacity. Lab Invest 30:1–8

94 Dantchev D (1978) Scanning electron microscopy morphology of mononuclear leucocytes in normal subjects and in patients with lymphoid and monocytoid neoplasias. Recent Results Cancer Res 64:94–107

95 Dao C, Marie JP, Bernadou A, Bilski-Pasquier G (1978) T-lymphocyte colonies in the lymphoproliferative disorders. Immunology 34:741–750

96 Davey RR, Dock NL, Wolos JA (to be published 1980) Studies of lymphocyte proliferation in hairy cell leukaemia: activity in mixed lymphocyte reaction and responses to mitogens. Br J Haematol

97 Davies GE, Wiernik PH (1977) Hairy cell leukemia with chylous ascites. JAMA 238:1541–1542

98 Davis AT, Brunning RD, Quie PG (1971) Polymorphonuclear leukocyte myeloperoxidase deficiency in a patient with myelomonocytic leukemia. N Engl J Med 285:789–791

99 Davis S (1976) The variable pattern of circulating lymphocyte subpopulations in chronic lymphocytic leukemia. N Engl J Med 294:1150–1153

100 Davis TE, Waterbury L, Abeloff M, Burke PJ (1976) Leukemic reticuloendotheliosis. Report of a case with prolonged remission following intensive chemotherapy. Arch Intern Med 136:620–622

101 Debusscher L, Bernheim JL, Collard-Ronge E, Govaerts A, Hooghe R, Lejeune FJ, Zeicher M, Strychmans PA (1975) Hairy cell leukemia: functional, immunologic, kinetic and ultrastructural characterization. Blood 46:495–507

102 Deegan MJ, Cossman J, Chosney BT, Schnitzer B (1976) Hairy cell leukemia. An immunologic and ultrastructural study. Cancer 38:1952–1961

103 Deiman W, Fahimi HD (1979) The appearance of transition forms between monocytes and Kupffer cells in the liver of rats treated with glucan. A cytochemical and ultrastructural study. J Exp Med 149:883–987

104 Delsol G, Pellegrin M, Corberand J, Guiu M, Pris J, Fabre J (1977) Hairy cell leukemia – a disease of the mononuclear phagocytes? In: Wisse E, Knook DL (eds) Kupffer cells and other liver sinusoidal cells. Elsevier/North Holland, Amsterdam

105 Dhaliwal HS, Ling NR, Bishop S, Chapel H (1978) Expression of immunoglobulin G on blood lymphocytes in chronic lymphocytic leukaemia. Clin Exp Immunol 31:226–236

106 Dickler HB (1974) Studies of the human lymphocyte receptor for heat-aggregated or antigen-complexed immunoglobulin. J Exp Med 140:508–522

107 Dickler HB (1976) Lymphocyte binding of aggregated immunoglobulin. Scand J Immunol [Suppl] 5:91–97

108 Dickler HB (1976) Studies of the association between Ia antigens and Fc receptors. In: Litwin SD, Christian CL, Siskind GW (eds) Clinical evaluation of immune function in man. Grune and Stratton, New York

109 Diebold J, Chomette G, Reynes M, Tricot G (1977) The spleen in hairy cell leukemia. Virchows Archiv [Pathol Anat] 372:325–336

110 Downey H (1938) Handbook of hematology, vol II. Hoeber, New York

111 Duhamel G (1971) Lymphoid myelofibrosis. About 10 further observations. Acta Haematol (Basel) 45:89–98

112 Düllmann J, Wulfhekel U, Drescher S, Hausmann K (1974) Die Haarzellenhämoblastose („hairy-cell leukemia"). Klinische, licht- und elektronenmikroskopische Befunde. Dtsch Med Wochenschr 99:859–863

113 El-Maalam H, Fletcher J (1976) Defective neutrophil function in chronic granulocytic leukaemia. Br J Haematol 34:95–103

114 Emberger JM, Navarro M, Rizkilla N, Izarn P (1973) Etude histologique et cytologique de la moelle osseuse et de la rate au cours de l'histiolymphocytose primitive médullaire et splénique. Nouv Rev Fr Hématol 13:365–375

115 Emberger J-M, Navarro M, Rizkalla N, Izarn P (1978) Splenic pseudosinuses, hepatic angiomatous lesions and hairy cell leukemia. Am J Clin Pathol 69:194

116 Ewald O (1923) Die leukämische Retikuloendotheliose. Dtsch Arch Klin Med 142:222–228

117 Fabre J, Delsol G, Fédou R, Pris J (1974) Etude des lésions hépatiques de la "Hairy Cell Leukemia". Virchows Archiv [Cell Pathol] 15:139–156

118 Fahimi JD (1978) The fine structural localization of endogenous and exogenous peroxidase activity in Kupffer cells of rat liver. J Cell Biol 47:247–262

119 Feiner AS, Myers AM, Moore GE (1978) Leukemic reticuloendotheliosis. Loss of platelet defect after splenectomy. JAMA 240:238–240

120 Fellons M, Hors MC, Rebourcet R, Finaz C, Weil D, Heuertz S, Wiels J, Mahouy G, Fridman WH (1977) The expression and relation of HLA, β2-microglobulin and receptor for marmoset red blood cells on man/mouse and man/Chinese hamster hybrid cells. Eur J Immunol 7:22–26

121 Ferrari GP, Uccella R (1977) Leukemic reticuloendotheliosis. Minerva Med 68:1727–1730

122 Ferrarini M, Hoffman T, Fu SM, Winchester R, Kunkel HG (1977) Receptors for IgM on certain human B lymphocytes. J Immunol 119:1525–1529

123 Fieschi A (1942) Istioleucemia (Retoteliosi leucemica). Haematologica (Paris) 24:751–774

124 Flandrin G, Ripault J (1969) Histio-lymphocytose médullaire et splénique de l'adulte. Etude de 19 cas. Actual Hematol 3:18–29

125 Flandrin G, Daniel MT, Fourcade M, Chelloul N (1973) Leucémie à "tricholeucocyte" (hairy cell leukemia). Étude clinique et cytologique de 55 observations. Nouv Rev Fr Hématol 13:609–640

126 Foa R, Catovsky D (1979) T-lymphocyte colonies in normal blood, bone marrow and lymphoproliferative disorders. Clin Exp Immunol 36:488–495

127 Foadi MD, Slater AM, Pegrum GD (1978) Erythrophagocytosis by acute lymphoblastic leukaemic cells. Scand J Haematol 20:85–88

128 Froland SS, Natvig JB (1973) Identification of three different human lymphocyte subpopulations by surface markers. Transplant Rev 16:114–162

129 Fu SM, Winchester RJ, Rai KR, Kunkel HG (1974) Hairy cell leukemia: proliferation of a cell with phagocytic and B-lymphocyte properties. Scand J Immunol 3:847–851

130 Fu SM, Chiorazzi N, Kunkel HG, Halper JP, Harris SR (1978) Induction of of in vitro differentiation and immunoglobulin synthesis of human leukemic B lymphocytes. J Exp Med 148:1570–1578

131 Furusawa S (1976) Hairy cell leukemia of B-lymphocyte nature: Demonstration of monoclonal surface IgG. Acta Haematol Jpn 39:767–771

132 Fuson EW, Whitten HD, Ayers RD, Lamon EW (1978) Antibody-dependent cell-mediated cytotoxicity by human lymphocytes. I. Comparison of IgM- and IgG-induced cytotoxicity. J Immunol 120:1726–1732

133 Gahmberg CG, Andersson LC (1978) Identification and characterization of normal and malignant human blood leukocytes by surface glycoprotein patterns. Ann NY Acad Sci 312:240–255

134 Galton DAG, Goldman JM, Wiltshaw E, Catovsky D, Henry K, Goldenberg GJ (1974) Prolymphocytic leukaemia. Br J Haematol 27:7–23

135 Gardner FH, Pringle JC Jr. (1961) Androgens and erythropoiesis 1. Preliminary clinical observations. Arch Intern Med 107:846–862

136 Garrett JV, Newton RK, Scarffe JH (1977) Abnormal blood lymphocytes in non-Hodgkin's lymphoma. Lancet 1:542

137 Garrett JV, Scarffe JH, Newton RK (1979) Abnormal peripheral blood lymphocytes and bone marrow infiltration in non-Hodgkin's lymphoma. Br J Haematol 42:41–50

138 Gathings WE, Lawton AR, Cooper MD (1977) Immunofluorescent studies of the development of pre-B cells, B lymphocytes and immunoglobulin isotype diversity in humans. Eur J Immunol 7:804–810

139 Ghadially FN, Skinnider LF (1972) Ultrastructure of hairy cell leukemia. Cancer 29:444–452

140 Gladkowska-Dura MJ, Wozniewicz BM, Dura WT (1977) An ultrastructural study of "hairy cell" leukemia (HCL) Acta Med Pol 18:317–318

141 Golde DW, Quan SG, Cline MJ (1976) Hairy cell leukemia: in-vitro culture studies. Ann Intern Med 85:78–79

142 Golde DW, Quan SG, Cline MJ (1978) Human T lymphocyte cell line producing colony-stimulating activity. Blood 52:1068–1072

143 Golde DW, Saxon A, Stevens RH (1977) Macroglobulinaemia and hairy cell leukemia. N Engl J Med 296:92–93

144 Golde DW, Stevens RH, Quan SG, Saxon A (1977) Immunoglobulin synthesis in hairy cell leukaemia. Br J Haematol 35:359–365

145 Goldstone AH, Cawley JC, Hayhoe FGJ (1976) Leukaemia, lymphoma and allied disorders. Saunders, London

146 Golomb HM (1978) Hairy cell leukemia: an unusual lymphoproliferative disease. A study of 24 patients. Cancer 42:946–956

146a Golomb HM, Mintz U (1979) Treatment of hairy cell leukemia (leukemic reticuloendotheliosis). II. Chlorambucil therapy in postsplenectomy patients with progressive disease. Blood 54:305–309

147 Golomb HM, Simon D (1977) Hairy-cell leukaemia. Lancet 1:372–373

148 Golomb HM, Braylan R, Polliack A (1975) Hairy cell leukemia (leukemic reticuloendotheliosis): a scanning electron microscopic study of eight cases. Br J Haematol 29:453–458

149 Golomb HM, Catovsky D, Golde DW (1978) Hairy cell leukemia. Ann Intern Med 89:677–683

150 Golomb HM, Lindgren V, Rowley JD (1978) Chromosome abnormalities in patients with hairy cell leukemia. Cancer 41:1374–1380

151 Golomb HM, Vardiman J, Sweet DL, Simon D, Variakojis D (1978) Hairy-cell leukaemia: evidence for the existence of a spectrum of functional characteristics. Br J Haematol 38:161–170

152 Gonzales-Molina A, Spiegelberg HL (1977) A subpopulation of normal human peripheral B lymphocytes that bind IgE. J Clin Invest 59:616–624

153 Gooi J, Burns GF, Cawley JC (1979) Hairy-cell leukaemia: an immunoperoxidase study of parafin-embedded tissues. J Clin Pathol 32:1244–1247

154 Gordon J, Smith JL (1978) Free immunoglobulin light chain synthesis by neoplastic cells in leukaemic reticuloendotheliosis. Clin Exp Immunol 31:244–250

155 Gordon J, Smith JL, Roath S (1978) Free immunoglobulin light chain synthesis by neoplastic cells from six cases of leukaemic reticuloendotheliosis. Br J Haematol 37:150

156 Gordon J, Hough D, Karpas A, Smith JL (1977) Immunoglobulin expression and synthesis by human haemic cells. Immunology 32:559–565

157 Gosselin GR, Hanlon DG, Pease GL (1956) Leukaemic reticuloendotheliosis. Can Med Assoc J 74:886–891

158 Gourdin MF, Reyes F, Lejonc JL, Mannoni P, Dreyfus B (1976) Surface features of cells in human lymphoproliferative disorders. An immunoelectron microscopy study. Haematol Bluttrans 19:207–219

159 Graham RC, Bernier GM (1975) The bone marrow in multiple myeloma: correlation of plasma cell ultrastructure and clinical state. Medicine (Baltimore) 54:225–243

160 Greaves MF, Janossy G (1976) Anti-human T cell sera. In: Bloom B, David J (eds) In vitro methods in cell mediated and tumor immunity. Academic Press, New York

161 Grossi CE, Webb SR, Zicca A, Lydyard PM, Moretta L, Mingari MC, Cooper MD (1978) Morphological and histochemical analysis of two human T-cell subpopulations bearing receptors for IgM or IgG. J Exp Med 147:1405–1417

162 Gupta S, Good RA, Siegal FP (1976) Rosette-formation with mouse erytrhocytes. II. A marker for human B and non-T lymphocytes. Clin Exp Immunol 25:319–327

163 Gupta S, Pahwa R, O'Reilly R, Good RA, Siegal FP (1976) Ontogeny of lymphocyte subpopulations in human fetal liver. Proc Natl Acad Sci USA 73:919

164 Haak HL, de Man JCH, Hijmans W, Knapp Q, Speck B (1974) Further evidence for the lymphocytic nature of leukaemic reticuloendotheliosis (hairy-cell leukaemia). Br J Haematol 27:31–38

165 Haegert DG, Hurd C, Coombs RRA (1978) Comparison of the direct antiglobulin rosetting reaction with direct immunofluorescence in the detection of surface membrane immunoglobulin on human peripheral blood lymphocytes. Immunology 34:533–538

166 Haegert DG, Cawley JC, Collins RD, Flemans RJ, Smith JL (1974) Leukaemic reticuloendotheliosis: a morphological and immunological study of four cases. J Clin Pathol 27:967–972

167 Hahner U, Burkhardt R (1977) Knochenmarksdiagnostik bei Haarzell-Leukämie. Klin Wochenschr 55:933–944

168 Harker WG, Rothstein G, Clarkson D, Athens JW, Macfarlane JL (1977) Enhancement of colony-stimulating activity production by lithium. Blood 49:263–267

169 Hartmann D, Obrecht JP, Gudat F, Hess M, Duvig P, Nissen C, Schmidt R, Pietra CD (1978) Besonderheiten der Haarzell-Leukämie. Schweiz Med Wochenschr 108:962–965

170 Hayhoe FGJ, Quaglino D, Doll R (1964) The cytology and cytochemistry of acute leukaemias. A study of 140 cases. MRC Special Report Series Number 304. Her Majesty's Stationary Office, London

171 Hayhoe FGJ, Flemans RJ, Burns GF, Cawley JC (1977) Leucocyte alkaline phosphatase scores in hairy cell leukaemia. Br J Haematol 37:158–159

172 Hayward AR, Layward L, Lydyard PM, Moretta L, Dagg M, Lawton AR (1978) Fc-receptor heterogeneity of human suppressor T cells. J Immunol 121:1–5

173 Hendrick AM, Hendrick DJ (1979) Scotochromogen infection in hairy-cell leukaemia. Lancet 1:109–110

174 Hernandez D, Cruz C, Carnot J, Dorticos E, Espinosa E (1978) Hairy cell leukaemia of T-cell origin. Br J Haematol 40:504–506

175 Heyden v HW, Waller HD, Pape GB, Benöhr HChr, Braun HJ, Wilms K, Rieber EP, Riethmüller G (1976) Haarzell-Leukämie. I. Klinik, Zytochemie, Phagozyosefähigkeit von Haarzellen, Etablierung permanent wachsender Zellinien. Dtsch Med Wochenschr 101:3–8

176 Higgy KE, Burns GF, Hayhoe FGJ (1977) Discrimination of B, T and null lymphocytes by esterase cytochemistry. Scand J Haematol 18:437–448

177 Higgy KE, Burns GF, Hayhoe FGJ (1978) Identification of the hairy cells of leukemic reticuloendotheliosis by an esterase method. Br J Haematol 38:99–106

178 Horwitz DA, Garrett MA (1977) Distinctive functional properties of human blood L lymphocytes: a comparison with T lymphocytes, B lymphocytes, and monocytes. J Immunol 118:1712–1721
179 Horwitz DA, Lobo PI (1975) Characterization of two populations of human lymphocytes bearing easily detectable surface immunoglobulin. J Clin Invest 56:1464–1472
180 Hoshino M (1969) Polysome-lamellae complex in the adenoma cells of the human adrenal cortex. J Ultrastruct Res 27:205–215
181 Hsu CCS, Marti GE, Schrek R, Williams RC (1975) Lymphocytes bearing B- and T-cell markers in patient with lymphosarcoma cell leukemia. Clin Immunol Immunopathol 3:385–395
182 Huber C, Asamer H, Michlmayr G, Braunsteiner H (1976) Surface immunoglobulins and receptor sites for aggregated IgG on leukemic reticuloendotheliosis cells. Blut 32:21–28
183 Hughes GRV, Elkon KB, Spiller R, Catovsky D, Jamieson I (1979) Polyarteritis nodosa and hairy-cell leukaemia. Lancet 1:678
184 Inoue T, Kubo S, Saitoh Y, Furusawa S, Tanaka Y (1976) Hairy cell leukemia: alterations of SEM images by preparation timing. J Clin Electron Micros 9:643
185 Jaffe ES, Shevach EM, Frank MM, Green I (1974) Leukemic reticuloendotheliosis: presence of a receptor for cytophilic antibody. Am J Med 57:108–114
186 James V (1978) Stereological analyses of leukaemic cells. Br J Haematol 39:17–24
187 Janckila AJ, Yam LT (1979) Cytochemistry of tartrate-resistant acid phosphatase. Am J Clin Pathol 71:356–357
188 Janckila AJ, Li CY, Lam KW, Yam LT (1978) The cytochemistry of tartrate-resistant acid phosphatase. Technical considerations. Am J Clin Pathol 70:45–55
189 Jansen J, Hermans J, Remme J, den Ottolander GJ, Lopes Cardoza P (1978) Hairy cell leukaemia. Clinical features and effect of splenectomy. Scand J Haematol 21:60–71
190 Jansen J, Schuit HRE, Schreuder GMTh, Muller HP, Meijer CJLM (1979) Distinct subtype within the spectrum of hairy cell leukemia. Blood 54:459–467
191 Jansen J, Schuit HRE, van Zwet ThL, Meijer CJLM, Hijmans W (1979) Hairy-cell leukaemia: a B-lymphocytic disorder. Br J Haematol 42:21–33
192 Jansen J, Meijer CJLM, van der Valk P, de Bruijn WC, Leijh PCJ, den Ottolander GJ, van Furth R (1979) Phagocytic potential of hairy cells. Scand J Haematol 23:69–79
193 Jayaswal U, Roath S, Hyde RD, Chisholm DM, Smith JL (1977) Blood lymphocyte surface markers and clinical findings in chronic lymphoproliferative disorders. Br J Haematol 37:207–215
194 Jondal M, Klein G, Oldstone MBA, Bokish V, Yefenof E (1976) Surface markers on human B and T lymphocytes. VIII. Association between complement and Epstein-Barr virus receptors on human lymphoid cells. Scand J Immunol 5:401–410
195 Joshi JH, Robinson WA, Charan NB, Mathew M (1977) Leukemic reticuloendotheliosis (hairy cell leukemia). J Assoc Physicians India 25:933–937
196 Kaplan J, Shope TC, Peterson WD (1974) Epstein-Barr virus-negative human malignant T-cell lines. J Exp Med 139:1070–1076
197 Kaplan ME, Clark C (1974) An improved rosetting assay for detection of human T lymphocytes. J Immunol Methods 5:131–135
198 Karpas A, Hayhoe FGJ, Greenberger JS, Barker CR, Cawley JC, Lowenthal RM, Maloney WC (1977) The establishment and cytological, cytochemical and immunological characterisation of human haemic cell lines: evidence for heterogeneity. Leukemia Res 1:35–49
199 Kass L (1977) Nonspecific esterase activity in 'hairy cells'. Acta Haematol (Basel) 58:103–107
200 Kass L, Schnitzer B (1973) Monocytes, monocytosis and monocytic leukemia. Thomas, Springfield, Ill.
201 Katayama I (1977) Hairy cell leukemia. N Engl J Med 296:881
202 Katayama I, Finkel HE (1974) Leukemic reticuloendotheliosis. A clinicopathologic study with review of the literature. Am J Med 57:115–126

203 Katayama I, Schneider GB (1977) Further ultrastructural characterization of hairy cells of leukemic reticuloendotheliosis. Am J Pathol 86:163–174

204 Katayama I, Yang JP (1977) Reassessment of a cytochemical test for differential diagnosis of leukemic reticuloendotheliosis. Am J Clin Pathol 68:268–272

205 Katayama I, Li CY, Yam LT (1972) Histochemical study of acid phosphatase isoenzyme in leukemic reticuloendotheliosis. Cancer 29:157–164

206 Katayama I, Li CY, Yam LT (1972) Ultrastructural characteristics of the 'hairy cells' of leukemic reticuloendotheliosis. Am J Pathol 67:361–370

207 Katayama I, Li CY, Yam LT (1972) Ultrastructural cytochemical demonstration of tartrate-resistant acid phosphatase isoenzyme activity in 'hairy cells' of leukemic reticuloendotheliosis. Am J Pathol 69:471–477

208 Katayama I, Nagy GK, Balogh K (1973) Light microscopic identification of the ribosome-lamella complex in 'hairy cells' of leukemic reticuloendotheliosis. Cancer 32:843–846

209 Kaufman S, Hergzeg E, Geltner L, Leiba H (1971) Un cas de myélose lymphoide. Nouv Rev Fr Hématol 11:609–616

210 Keusch F, Ruttner JR, Pedio G, Gut D (1976) Occurrence of plasmocytoid cells in long-term blood-cell cultures from a patient with 'hairy cell' leukemia. Exp Cell Biol 44:20–27

211 King GW, Hurtubise PE, Sagone AL Jr, Lo Buglio AF, Metz EN (1975) Leukemic reticuloendotheliosis. A study of the origin of the malignant cell. Am J Med 59:411–416

212 Kingston P (1979) Personal communication. Pathology Department, Gloucester Royal Hospital, Great Western Road, Gloucester GL1 3NN

213 Kitani T (1976) Hairy cell leukemia. Studies on the nature of hairy cells. Acta Haematol Jpn 39:756–766

214 Kitani T (1976) Hairy cell leukemia. Studies on the nature of hairy cells with special reference to anti-hairy cell serum. Jpn J Clin Hematol 17:436–443

215 Kitani T (1977) Characterization of an anti-hairy cell serum. In: Seno S, Takaku F, Irino S (eds) Topics in haematology. Excerpta Medica, Amsterdam

216 Kjeldsberg CR (1978) Leukocyte mobilization in leukemic reticuloendotheliosis. Ann Intern Med 88:268–269

217 Komiyama A, Ogawa M, Eurenius K, Spicer SS (1976) Unusual cytoplasmic inclusions in blast cells in the acute leukemia. Arch Pathol Lab Med 100:590–594

218 Kramers MTC, Catovsky D, Foa R, Cherchi M, Galton DAG (1976) 5^1 nucleotidase activity in leukaemic lymphocytes. Biomedicine [Express] 25:363–365

219 Krause JR, Dekker A (1978) Hairy cell leukemia (leukemic reticuloendotheliosis) in serous effusions. Acta Cytol (Baltimore) 22:80–82

220 Krause JR, Nitiyanant P, Rabin BS (1978) Cryocrystalglobulinemia in hairy cell leukemia. Cancer 42:2798–2801

221 Krause JR, Srodes C, Lee RE (1977) Use of the bone marrow imprint in the diagnosis of leukemic reticuloendotheliosis ('hairy cell leukemia'). Am J Clin Pathol 68:368–371

222 Kuntz MM, Innes JB, Weksler ME (1976) Lymphocyte transformation induced by autologous cells. IV. Human T-lymphocyte proliferation induced by autologous or allogeneic non-T lymphocytes. J Exp Med 143:1042–1054

223 Lam KW, Dekker PT, Castleman J, Yam LT (1976) Studies of intracellular distribution of acid phosphatase 5 in the spleen cells of leukemic reticuloendotheliosis by isopycnic gradient centrifugation. Clin Chim Acta 70:289–295

224 Lam KW, Lai LC, Burkart PT, Yam LT (1977) Kinetic properties of tartrate-resistant acid phosphatase isolated from human spleen with leukemic reticuloendotheliosis. J Biol Chem 252:3371–3373

225 Leder LD (1978) Alkaline phosphatase and tartrate resistant acid phosphatase activity in cells of prolymphocytic leukemia. Klin Wochenschr 56:313–314

226 Lee SL, Rosner F, Rosenthal N, Rosenthal RL (1969) Reticulum cell leukemia. Clinical and hematologic entity. NY State J Med 69:422–429

227 Leech J, Roy RM, Flexner JM, Glick AD, Waldron JA, Collins RD (1975) Evidence for synthesis of surface immunoglobulin in leukemic reticuloendotheliosis. Blood 46: 1037
228 Leitner SJ (1949) Bone marrow biopsy. Haematology in the light of sternal puncture. Churchill, London
229 Lemon SM, Pagano JS, Utsinger PD, Sinkovics JG (1979) Cultured "hairy cells" infected with Epstein-Barr virus: evidence for B-lymphocyte origin. Ann Intern Med 90:54–55
230 Lennert K, Stein H (1978) Personal points of view on the Kiel classification. Recent Results Cancer Res 64:31–37
231 Levine PH, Katayama I (1975) The platelet in leukemic reticuloendotheliosis. Functional and morphological evidence of a qualitative disorder. Cancer 36: 1353–1358
232 Levy R, Warnke R, Dorfman RF, Haimovich J (1977) The monoclonality of human B-cell lymphomas. J Exp Med 145: 1014–1028
233 Lewis SM, Catovsky D, Hows JM, Ardalan B (1977) Splenic red cell pooling in hairy cell leukaemia. Br J Haematol 35: 351–357
234 Li CY, Yam LT, Lam KW (1970) Acid phosphatase isoenzyme in human leukocytes in normal and pathologic conditions. J Histochem Cytochem 18:473–481
235 Li CY, Yam LT, Lam KW (1970) Studies of acid phosphatase isoenzymes in human leukocytes. Demonstration of isoenzyme cell specificity. J Histochem Cytochem 18:901–910
236 Li CY, Lam KW, Yam LT (1973) Esterases in human leukocytes. J Histochem Cytochem 21:1–12
237 Ling NR, Bishop S, Jefferis R (1977) Use of antibody-coated red cells for the sensitive detection of antigen and in rosette tests for cells bearing surface immunoglobulins. J Immunol Methods 15:279–289
238 Lobo PL, Horwitz DA (1976) An appraisal of Fc receptors of human peripheral blood B and L lymphocytes. J Immunol 117:939–943
239 LoBuglio AF (1976) Leukemic reticuloendotheliosis: a defined syndrome of an ill defined cell. N Engl J Med 295:219–220
240 LoBuglio AF, Cottran RS, Jandl JH (1967) Red cells coated with immunoglobulin G: binding and sphering by mononuclear cells in man. Science 158: 1582–1585
241 Loffler H, Graubner M, Desaga JF, Jung M (1977) Prolymphocytic leukemia with T cell properties and tartrate resistant acid phosphatase. In: Thierfelder S, Rodt H, Thiel E (eds) Immunological diagnosis of leukemias and lymphomas. Springer, Berlin Heidelberg New York
242 Lohrmann H-P, Novikov L (1974) Rosette formation between human T-lymphocytes and unsensitized rhesus monkey erythrocytes. Clin Immunol Immunopathol 3:99–111
243 Loor F (1977) Structure and dynamics of the lymphocyte surface. In: Loor F, Roelants GE (eds) B and T cells in immune recognition. Wiley, London
244 Lusch CJ, Ramsey HE, Katayama I (1978) Leukemic reticuloendotheliosis. Report of a case with peripheral blood remission on androgen therapy. Cancer 41: 1964–1966
245 Ly IA, Mishell RI (1974) Separation of mouse spleen cells by passage through columns of sephadex G-10. J Immunol Methods 5:239–247
246 Maino VC, Kurnick JT, Kubo RT, Grey HM (1977) Mitogen activation of human chronic lymphatic leukemia cells. 1. Synthesis and secretion of immunoglobulin. J Immunol 118:742–748
247 Manes JL, Blair OM (1976) Disseminated Mycobacterium kansasii infection complicating hairy cell leukemia. JAMA 236: 1878–1879
248 Marie JP, Degos L, Flandrin G (1977) Hairy cell leukemia and tuberculosis. N Engl J Med 297: 1354
249 Matre R, Talstad I, Haugen A (1977) Surface markers in non-phagocytic hairy cell leukemia. Acta Pathol Microbiol Scand [C] 85:406–412
250 McCarthy D, Catovsky D (1978) Response to doxorubicin in hairy cell leukaemia. Scand J Haematol 21:445–447

251 McConnell I, Hurd CM (1976) Lymphocyte receptors. II. Receptors for rabbit IgM on human T lymphocytes. Immunology 30:835–839

252 McKenna RW, Bloomfield CD, Dick F, Nesbit ME, Brunning RD (1975) Acute monoblastic leukemia: diagnosis and treatment of ten cases. Blood 46:481–494

253 Meier J, Coleman MS, Hutton JJ (1976) Adenosine deaminase activity in peripheral blood cells of patients with haematological malignancies. Br J Cancer 33:312–319

254 Meister H (1975) "Hairy cell"-Leukämie. Folia Haematol (Leipz) 102:634–638

255 Mellstedt M, Hammarström S, Holm G (1974) Monoclonal lymphocyte population in human plasma cell myeloma. Clin Exp Immunol 17:371–384

256 Mendes NF, Miki SS, Peixinho ZF (1974) Combined detection of human T and B lymphocytes by rosette formation with sheep erythrocytes and zymosan-C3 complexes. J Immunol 113:531–536

257 Metcalf D (1977) Hemopoietic colonies. Springer, Berlin Heidelberg New York

258 Mitus WJ, Mednicoff IB, Wittels B, Dameshek W (1961) Neoplastic lymphoid reticulum cells in the peripheral blood: a histochemical study. Blood 17:206–215

259 Miura AB (1976) Hairy cell leukemia: diagnostic criteria from the clinical point of view. Acta Haematol Jpn 39:705–713

260 Miyoshi I, Hiraki S, Hikita T, Ota T, Tsubota T, Tanaka T, Kimura I (1978) Hairy cell leukemia – transplantation into hamsters and production of tumours. Am J Clin Pathol 71:358–359

261 Möbius W, Hennekeuser HH, Westerhausen M, Stang-Voss G, Lesch R (1975) Haarzell-Leukämie. Acta Haematol (Basel) 53:1–16

262 Moretta L, Mingari MC, Romanzi CA (1978) Loss of Fc receptors for IgG from human T lymphocytes exposed to IgG immune complexes. Nature 272:618–620

263 Moretta L, Ferrarini M, Durante ML, Mingari MC (1975) Expression of a receptor for IgM by human T cells in vitro. Eur J Immunol 5:565–569

264 Moretta L, Mingari MC, Moretta A, Lydyard PM (1977) Receptors for IgM are expressed on acute lymphoblastic leukemic cells bearing T-cell characteristics. Clin Immunol Immunopathol 7:405–409

265 Moretta L, Ferrarini M, Mingari MC, Moretta A, Webb SR (1976) Subpopulations of human T cells identified by receptors for immunoglobulins and mitogen responsiveness. J Immunol 117:2171–2174

266 Moretta L, Webb SR, Grossi CE, Lydyard PM, Cooper MD (1977) Functional analysis of two human T-cell subpopulations: help and suppression of B-cell responses by T cells bearing receptors for IgM or IgG. J Exp Med 146:184–200

267 Mover S, Li CY, Yam LT (1972) Semiquantitative evaluation of tartrate-resistant acid phosphatase activity in human blood cells. J Lab Clin Med 80:711–717

268 Nabarra B, Sonsino E, Andrianarison I (1977) Ultrastructure of a polysome-lamellae complex in a human paraganglioma. Am J Pathol 86:523–532

269 Naeim F, Smith GS (1974) Leukemic reticuloendotheliosis. Cancer 34:1813–1821

270 Naeim F, Gossett T, Walford RL (1977) Reactivity of the Merrit B-cell alloantiserums with hairy cells. N Engl J Med 296:882

271 Naeim F, Capostagno VJ, Johnson CE Jr, Lehrer R, Gatti RA (1979) Sézary syndrome. Tartrate-resistant acid phosphatase in the neoplastic cells. Am J Clin Pathol 71:528–533

272 Naeim F, Gatti RA, Johnson CE, Gossett T, Walford RL (1978) "Hairy cell" leukemia. A heterogeneous chronic lymphoproliferative disorder. Am J Med 65:479–487

273 Najarian T, Colton T (1978) Mortality from leukaemia and cancer in shipyard nuclear workers. Lancet 1:1018–1020

274 Nanba K, Braylan RC (1976) Leukemic reticuloendotheliosis and 'hairy cells'. N Engl J Med 295:1015

275 Nanba K, Soban EJ, Bowling MC, Berard CW (1977) Splenic pseudosinuses and hepatic angiomatous lesions. Distinctive features of hairy cell leukemia. Am J Clin Pathol 67:415–426

276 Nanba K, Jaffe ES, Soban EJ, Braylan RC, Berard CW (1977) Hairy cell leukemia. Enzyme histochemical characterization, with special reference to splenic stromal changes. Cancer 39:2323–2336

277 Nath I, Curtis J, Mangalik A, Talwar GP (1975) Lymphocytes devoid of T and B cell markers in chronic lymphatic leukemia. Acta Haematol (Basel) 53:37–43

278 Natvig JB, Froland SS (1976) Detection of a third lymphocyte-like cell type by rosette formation with erythrocytes sensitised by various anti-Rh antibodies. Scand J Immunol [Suppl] 5:83–89

279 Neiman RS, Sullivan AL, Jaffe R (1979) Malignant lymphoma simulating leukemic reticuloendotheliosis. Cancer 43:329–342

280 Novikoff AB, Goldfischer S (1968) Visualization of microbodies for light and electron microscopy. J Histochem Cytochem 16:507

281 Ohtsuki Y, Dmochowski L, Seman G, Bowen JM, Johnson DE (1978) Particle-lamella complexes in a case of human benign prostate hyperplasia. J Natl Cancer Inst 60:299–302

282 O'Riordan ML, Berry EW, Tough IM (1970) Chromosome studies on bone marrow from a male control population. Br J Haematol 19:83–90

283 Padilla F, Soloff BL (1969) Electron microscopic observations on "hairy" lymphoreticular cells. Clin. Res 17b:32

284 Padilla F, Soloff BL (1971) Leukemic reticuloendotheliosis. Electron microscopy of circulating lymphoid cells. Nouv Rev Fr Hématol 11:547–554

285 Palutke M, Tabaczka P (1979) Functional studies of hairy cell leukemia (leukemic reticuloendotheliosis). Am J Clin Pathol 7:273–280

286 Palutke M, Weise RW, Tabaczka P, Varadachari C, Axelrod A (1978) Hairy cells and macrophages. A comparative study. Lab Invest 39:267–280

287 Pareti FI, Capitano A, Mannucci PM (1976) Acquired storage pool disease in platelets during disseminated intravascular coagulation. Blood 48:511–515

288 Parker AC, Stuart AE (1978) Ultrastructural studies of leucocytes which form rosettes with homologous erythrocytes in human autoimmune haemolytic anaemia. Scand J Haematol 20:129–140

289 Pedio G, Rüttner JR, Spycher MA, Gut D (1975) Virus-bearing plasma cells in peripheral blood of a patient with 'hairy cell' leukemia. Acta Haematol (Basel) 54:297–305

290 Pellegrino MA, Ferrone S, Theofilopoulos AN (1975) Rosette formation of human lymphoid cells with monkey red blood cells. J Immunol 115:1065–1071

291 Perlmann H, Perlmann P, Pape GR, Hallden G (1976) Purification, fractionation and assay of antibody-dependent lymphocyte effector cells (K cells) in human blood. Scand J Immunol [Suppl] 5:57–68

292 Pichler WJ, Broder S (1978) Fc-IgM and Fc-IgG receptors on human circulating B lymphocytes. J Immunol 121:887–890

293 Pichler WJ, Knapp W (1977) Receptors for IgM-coated erythrocytes on chronic lymphatic leukemia cells. J Immunol 118:1010–1015

294 Pichler WJ, Knapp W (1978) Receptors for IgM on human B lymphocytes. Scand J Immunol 7:105–109

295 Pichler WJ, Lum L, Broder S (1978) Fc-receptors on human T lymphocytes. I. Transition of Tγ to Tμ cells. J Immunol 121:1540–1548

296 Pierre RV, Hoagland HC (1972) Age-associated aneuploidy: loss of Y chromosome from human bone marrow cells with ageing. Cancer 30:889–894

297 Pinkus GS, Said JW (1977) Profile of intracytoplasmic lysozyme in normal tissues, myeloproliferative disorders, hairy cell leukemia, and other pathologic processes. An immunoperoxidase study of paraffin sections and smears. Am J Pathol 89:351–366

298 Plenderleith IH (1970) Hairy cell leukemia. Can Med Assoc J 102:1056–1060

299 Polliack A (1977) Normal, transformed and leukemic leukocytes. Springer, Berlin Heidelberg New York

300 Polliack A (1977) Surface morphology of leukemic cells: application of scanning electron microscopy to the study of human leukemias. Israel J Med Sci 13:701–710

301 Polliack A (1978) Surface morphology of lymphoreticular cells: review of data obtained from scanning electron microscopy. Recent Results Cancer Res 64:66–93

302 Polliack A, Braylan R, Golomb H (1974) Scanning electron microscopy of hairy cells in hairy-cell leukaemia. Lancet 2:1013–1014

303 Pozner LH, Daniels CA, Cooper JA, Cohen HJ, Logue GL, Croker BP (1978) Replication of type 1 Herpes simplex virus in primary cultures of hairy cell leukemic leukocytes. Am J Pathol 90:187–200

304 Preud'homme JL, Seligmann M (1972) Surface bound immunoglobulins as a cell marker in human lymphoproliferative diseases. Blood 40:777–794

305 Preud'homme JL, Seligmann M (1974) Surface immunoglobulins on human lymphoid cells. In: Schwartz RS (ed) Progress in clinical immunology. Grune and Stratton, New York

306 Preud'homme JL, Brouet JC, Seligmann M (1975) Lymphocyte membrane markers in human lymphoproliferative disease. In: Preud'homme JL, Kourilsky FM (eds) Membrane receptors of lymphocytes. North Holland, Amsterdam

307 Preud'homme JL, Brouet JC, Seligmann M (1977) Membrane-bound IgD on human lymphoid cells with special reference to immunodeficiency and immunoproliferative diseases. Immunol Rev 37:127–151

308 Rabinowitz Y, Schrek R (1962) "Monocytic" cells of normal blood, Schilling and Naegeli leukemia and leukemic reticuloendotheliosis in slide chambers. Blood 20:453–470

309 Revesz T, Greaves MF, Capellaro D, Murray RK (1976) Differential expression of cell surface binding sites for cholera toxin in acute and chronic leukaemias. Br J Haematol 34:623–630

310 Reyes F, Gourdin MF, Farcet JP, Dreyfus B (1976) Critères morphologiques de surfaces étudiés en microscopie électronique et classification des syndromes lymphoprolifératifs. Étude critique. Ann Méd Interne (Paris) 127:865–872

311 Reyes F, Gourdin MF, Farcet JP, Dreyfus B, Breton-Gorius J (1977) The presence of endogenous peroxidase activity in hairy cell leukemia. CR Acad Sci [D] (Paris) 284:493–496

312 Reyes F, Gourdin MF, Farcet JP, Dreyfus B, Breton-Gorius J (1978) Synthesis of a peroxidase activity by cells of hairy cell leukemia: a study by ultrastructural cytochemistry. Blood 52:537–550

313 Rhyner K, Streuli R, Kistler GS (1977) Hairy cell leukemia with osteolytic bone changes. Schweiz Med Wochenschr 107:863–871

314 Rieber EP, Heyden v HW, Linke RP, Saal JG, Riethmüller G, Waller HD (1976) Haarzell-Leukämie. Charakterisierung der leukämischen Zelle: Oberflächenimmunglobuline, Fc-Rezeptoren und Stimulation durch Mitogene. Klin Wochenschr 54:1011–1019

315 Rieber EP, Hadam MR, Linke RP, Saal JG, Riethmüller G, Heyden v HW, Waller HD (1979) Hairy cell leukaemia: surface markers and functional capacities of the leukaemic cells analysed in eight patients. Br J Haematol 42:175–188

316 Rieber EP, Linke RP, Hadam MR, Saal JG, Riethmüller G, Heyden v HW, Waller HD, Schwarz H (1977) Hairy cell leukaemia: simultaneous demonstration of autochthonous surface-Ig and monocytic functions of hairy cells. In: Thierfelder S, Rodt H, Thiel E (eds) Immunological diagnosis of leukemias and lymphomas. Springer, Berlin Heidelberg New York

317 Roath S, Newell DG (1975) Cell-surface characteristics in hairy-cell leukaemia. Lancet 1:283–284

318 Romagnani S, Maggi E, Biagiotti R, Giudizi GM, Amadori A, Ricci M (1978) Receptors for IgM: a feature of subpopulations of both T and B human lymphocytes. Clin Exp Immunol 32:324–332

319 Rosenthal N, Lee SL (1951) Reticulum cell leukemia: a clinical and morphologic entity. Report of 16 cases. Presented at the 13th Annual Meeting of the American Society of Clinical Pathologists, Chicago, October 16–19, 1951

320 Rosier RP, Lefer LG (1977) Spontaneous rupture of the spleen in hairy cell leukemia. Arch Pathol Lab Med 101:557

321 Ross GD, Polley MJ, Rabellino EM, Grey HM (1973) Two different complement receptors on human lymphocytes. One specific for C3b and one specific for C3b inactivator-cleaved C3b. J Exp Med 138:798–811

322 Rozenszajn LA, Gutman A, Radnay J, David EB, Shoham D (1976) A study of the nature of 'hairy' cells, with emphasis on enzymatic markers. Am J Clin Pathol 66:432–441

323 Rozman C, Woessner S (1978) Caracterización de la tricoleucemia por medio de la microscopia electrónica cuantitativa. Sangre 23:303–313

324 Rubin AD, Havemann K, Dameshek W (1969) Studies in chronic lymphocytic leukemia: further studies of the proliferative abnormality of the blood lymphocyte. Blood 33:313–328

325 Rubin AD, Douglas SD, Chessin LN, Glade PR, Dameshek W (1969) Chronic reticulolymphocytic leukemia. Reclassification of 'leukemic reticuloendotheliosis' through functional characterization of the circulating mononuclear cells. Am J Med 47:149–162

326 Ryser J-E, Vassalli P (1974) Mouse bone marrow lymphocytes and their differentiation. J Immunol 113:719–728

327 Salsano F (1978) Monoclonal immunoglobulins on the membrane of chronic lymphocytic leukaemia, hairy-cell leukaemia and non-Hodgkin's lymphoma cells. In: Ricci M, Fauci AS, Arcangeli P, Torzuoli P (eds) Developments in clinical immunology. Academic Press, London

328 Salsano F, Pisarri-Salsano S, Ciancarelli MP, Piantelli MP, Lauriola L, Musiani P (1979) Structural and functional characteristics of hairy cells. Acta Haematol (Basel) 61:184–193

329 Sanel FT, Serpick AA (1970) Plasmalemmal and subsurface complexes in human leukemic cells: membrane bonding by zipperlike junctions. Science 168:1458–1460

330 Saxon A, Stevens RH, Golde DW (1978) T-lymphocyte variant of hairy-cell leukemia. Ann Intern Med 88:323–326

331 Saxon A, Stevens RH, Quan SG, Golde DW (1978) Immunologic characterization of hairy cell leukemias in continuous cultures. J Immunol 120:777–782

332 Schaefer HE, Hellriegel KP, Zach J, Fischer R (1975) Zytochemischer Polymorphismus der sauren Phosphatase bei Haarzell-Leukämie. Blut 31:365–370

333 Scheinberg M, Brenner AI, Sullivan AL, Cathcart ES, Katayama I (1976) The heterogeneity of leukemic reticuloendotheliosis, 'hairy-cell leukaemia'. Evidence for its monocytic origin. Cancer 37:1302–1307

334 Schlossman SF, Chess L (1976) Immunologic functions of a subset of human null cells. In: Litwin SD, Christian CL, Siskind GW (eds) Clinical evaluation of immune function in man. Grune and Stratton, New York

335 Schmalzl F, Huhn D, Asamer H, Braunsteiner H (1975) Hairy cell leukemia ('leukemic reticuloendotheliosis'), reticulosarcoma, and monocytic leukemia. Cytochemical and ultrastructural investigations. Acta Haematol (Basel) 53:257–276

336 Schnitzer B, Hammack WJ (1974) B-lymphocyte nature of hairy cells in hairy-cell leukaemia. Lancet 2:649

337 Schnitzer B, Kass L (1974) Hairy-cell leukemia. A clinicopathologic and ultrastructural study. Am J Clin Pathol 61:176–187

338 Schnitzer B, Mead ML (1975) Nature of the hairy cell. Lancet 1:805

339 Schrek R, Donnelly WJ (1966) 'Hairy' cells in blood in lymphoreticular neoplastic disease and 'flagellated' cells of normal lymph nodes. Blood 27:199–211

340 Sebahoun G, Boufette P, Flandrin G (1978) Hairy cell leukemia. Leukemia Res 2:187–195

341 Seligmann M (1977) Discussion of: Surface receptors of human neoplastic lymphoreticular cells. In: Thierfelder S, Rodt H, Thiel E (eds) Immunological diagnosis of leukemias and lymphomas. Springer, Berlin Heidelberg New York

342 Seshadri RS, Brown EJ, Zipursky A (1976) Leukemic reticuloendotheliosis. A failure of monocyte production. N Engl J Med 295:181–184
343 Shevach EM, Jaffe ES, Green I (1973) Receptors for complement and immunoglobulin on human and animal lymphoid cells. Transplant Rev 16:3–28
344 Siegal FP, Good RA (1977) Human lymphocyte differentiation markers and their application to immune deficiency and lymphoproliferative diseases. Clin Haematol 6:355–422
345 Sinkovics JG, Györkey F, Györkey P (1976) Leukemic reticuloendotheliosis and 'hairy cells'. N Engl J Med 295:1016
346 Sinkovics JG, Wang C-H, Györkey F (1975) Hairy cells in culture. Lancet 1:749–750
347 Sinkovics JG, Györkey F, Györkey P, Wang C-H (1976) Hairy cells in long-term cultures. Ann Intern Med 85:532–533
348 Slater NGP, Barkhan P, Williams HJH (1979) Hairy cell leukaemia – apparent cure with reversal of marrow fibrosis. Clin Lab Haematol 1:65–68
349 Smith JB, Knowlton RP, Koons IS (1977) Immunologic studies in chronic lymphocytic leukemia: defective stimulation of T-cell proliferation in autologous mixed lymphcyte culture. J Natl Cancer Inst 58:579–585
350 Smith WI, Zidar BL, Winkelstein A, Whiteside TL, Shadduck RK, Zeigler Z, Brietfeld V, Silverberg JH, Rosenback LM, Rabin BS (1977) Hairy cell leukemia. A case with B-lymphocyte origin. Am J Clin Pathol 68:778–786
351 Solheim BG, Thorsby E, Möller E (1976) Inhibition of the Fc receptor of human lymphoid cells by antisera-recognizing determinants of the HLA system. J Exp Med 143:1568–1574
352 Spiegelberg HL, Dainer PM (1979) Fc receptors for IgG, IgM and IgE on human leukaemic lymphocytes. Clin Exp Immunol 35:286–295
353 Sprent J (1977) Migration and lifespan of lymphocytes. In: Loor F, Roelants GE (eds) B and T cells in immune recognition. Wiley, London
354 Spriggs AI (1976) Hairy cells. Lancet 1:427
355 Springer TA, Kaufman JF, Giphart M, Mann DL, Terhorst C, Strominger J (1976) Chemical and immunological characterization of HLA-linked B-lymphocyte alloantigens. Cold Spring Harbor Symp Quant Biol 41:387–396
356 Srivastava BI, Khan SA, Song SY (1978) Terminal deoxynucleotidyl transferase in hairy-cell leukaemia and Hodgkin's disease. Br J Cancer 38:643
357 Stang-Voss C, Moebius M (1976) Zur Ultrastruktur des sogenannten Ribosomen-Lamellen-Komplexes bei Haarzell-Leukämie. Verh Anat Ges 70:931–938
358 Stass SA, Holloway ML, Slease RB, Schumacher HR (1977) Spurious platelet counts in hairy cell leukemia. Am J Clin Pathol 68:530
359 Stathopoulos G, Elliot EV (1974) Formation of mouse or sheep red-blood cell rosettes by lymphocytes from normal and leukaemic individuals. Lancet 2:600–601
360 Stefani S, Chandra S, Schrek R, Tonaki H, Knospe WH (1977) Endoplasmic reticulum-associated structures in lymphocytes from patients with chronic lymphocytic leukemia. Blood 50:125–139
361 Stein H, Kaiserling E (1974) Surface immunoglobulins and lymphocyte-specific surface antigens on leukaemic reticuloendotheliosis cells. Clin Exp Immunol 18:63–71
362 Stein RS, Beaman C, Ali MY, Hansen R, Jenkins DD, Jume HG (1977) Lithium carbonate attenuation of chemotherapy-induced neutropenia. N Engl J Med 297:430–431
363 Stingl G, Knapp W (1977) Characterization of neoplastic mononuclear cells on tissue sections. In: Thierfelder S, Rodt H, Thiel E (eds) Immunological diagnosis of leukemias and lymphomas. Springer, Berlin Heidelberg New York
364 Stuart AE, Dewar AE (1979) Properties of anti-hairy cell serum. Br J Haematol 41:163–168
365 Sultan C, Marquet M (1975) Colony-stimulating capacity of cells of hairy-cell leukaemia. Lancet 1:920
366 Symmers St C (1978) Systemic pathology. Churchill Livingstone, Edingburgh

367 Szaniawski W (1977) Electron microscopy in diagnosis of hairy cell leukemia (HCL). Acta Med Pol 18:391

368 Tani E, Higashi N (1972) Particle-lamella complex and lamellar crystalloid in human meningioma. J Ultrastruct Res 41:334–343

369 Tigges FJ, Heyden v HW, Waller HD (1977) Kulturverhalten weißer Blutzellen bei Patienten mit Haarzell-Leukämie in der Diffusionskammer. Blut 35:103–113

370 Toyama K (1976) Hairy cell leukaemia: in relation to allied disorders. Acta Haematol Jpn 39:732–755

371 Treves AJ, Heidelberger E, Feldman M, Kaplan HS (1978) In vitro sensitization of human lymphocytes against histiocytic lymphoma cell lines. II. Characterization of two different effector activities and of suppressor cells. J Immunol 121:86–90

372 Trubowitz S, Masek B, Frasca JM (1971) Leukemic reticuloendotheliosis. Blood 38:288–298

373 Turner A, Kjeldsberg CR (1978) Hairy cell leukemia: a review. Medicine 57:477–499

374 Turpin F, Lejeune F, Lortholary P (1976) Inclusions tubulaires dans les lymphocytes d'une leucémie à tricholeucocytes. Pathol Biol (Paris) 24:287–292

375 Utsinger PD, Yount WJ, Fuller CR, Logue MJ, Orringer EP (1977) Hairy cell leukemia: B-lymphocyte and phagocytic properties. Blood 49:19–27

376 Vykoupil KF, Thiele J, Georgii A (1976) Hairy cell leukemia. Bone marrow findings in 24 patients. Virchows Archiv Pathol 370:273–290

377 Webb DI (1977) Hairy cell leukemia: a review. Alaska Med 19:40–42

378 Weinstein RA, Gelmann E, Golomb HM (1978) Disseminated atypical mycobacterial infection in hairy-cell leukaemia. Lancet 2:1052–1053

379 Weisberg SI (1975) Urinary muramidase in hairy cell leukemia. N Engl J Med 293:150–151

380 Wenzel KL, Ichiki AT (1977) A subpopulation of T cells detected by AET-treated sheep erythrocytes. Clin Immunol Immunopathol 8:73–79

381 Willcox MB, Golde DW, Cline MJ (1976) Cytochemical reactions of human haematopoietic cells in liquid culture. J Histochem Cytochem 24:979–983

382 Winchester RJ, Fu SM (1976) Lymphocyte surface membrane immunoglobulin. Scand J Immunol [Suppl] 5:77–82

383 Woessner S, Rozman C (1976) Ribosome-lamellae complex in chronic lymphatic leukemia. Blut 33:23–28

384 Worman CP, Burns GF, Barker CR (1978) Evidence for the presence of a receptor for IgM on the pathological cells of Sézary's syndrome. Clin Exp Immunol 31:391–396

385 Yam LT, Chaudhry AA, Janckila AJ (1977) Impaired marrow granulocyte reserve and leukocyte mobilization in leukemic reticuloendotheliosis. Ann Intern Med 87:444–446

386 Yam LT, Li CY, Finkel HE (1972) Leukemic reticuloendotheliosis. The role of tartrate-resistant acid phosphatase in diagnosis and splenectomy in treatment. Arch Intern Med 130:248–256

387 Yam LT, Li CY, Lam KW (1971) Tartrate-resistant acid phosphatase isoenzyme in the reticulum cells of leukemic reticuloendotheliosis. N Engl J Med 284:357–360

388 Yam LT, Tavassoli M, Jacobs P (1975) Differential characterization of the "reticulum cell" in lymphoreticular neoplasms. Am J Clin Pathol 64:171–179

389 Yam LT, Castoldi GL, Garvey MB, Mitus WJ (1968) Functional, cytogenetic and cytochemical study of the leukemic reticulum cells. Blood 32:90–101

390 Yamashita K, Inagaki T (1976) Hairy cell leukemia with special references to the relation to allied disorders. From the pathological standpoint. Acta Haematol Jpn 39:714–731

391 Yefenof E, Klein G (1977) Membrane receptor stripping confirms the association between EBV receptors and complement receptors on the surface of human B lymphoma lines. Int J Cancer 20:347–352

392 Yodoi J, Ishizaka K (1979) Lymphocytes bearing Fc receptors for IgE. I. Presence of human and rat T lymphocytes with Fcε receptors. J Immunol 122:2577–2583

393 Yoshikawa H, Takayama H, Ishiguro J, Yamada K, Suenaga M (1975) A case of "chronic" leukemic reticuloendotheliosis with excellent response to chemotherapy. Jpn J Clin Hematol 16:1050–1058

394 Zahavi J, Marder VJ (1974) Acquired 'storage pool disease' of platelets associated with circulating antiplatelet antibodies. Am J Med 56:883–890

395 Zidar BL, Winkelstein A, Whiteside TL, Shadduck RK, Zeigler Z, Smith WI, Rabin BS, Krause JR, Lee RE (1977) Hairy cell leukaemia: seven cases with probable B-lymphocytic origin. Br J Haematol 37:455–465

396 Zucker-Franklin D (1963) Virus-like particles in the lymphocytes of a patient with chronic lymphocytic leukemia. Blood 21:509–512

397 Zuzel M, Cawley JC, Paton RC, Burns GF, McNicol GP (1979) Platelet function in hairy-cell leukaemia. J Clin Pathol 32:814–821

Subject Index

Recent Results in Cancer Research

Sponsored by the Swiss League against Cancer. Editor in Chief: P. Rentchnick, Genève

For information about Vols. 1–9, please contact your bookseller or Springer-Verlag

10 NELSON, R. S.: Radioactive Phosphorus in the Diagnosis of Gastrointestinal Cancer.
11 FREEMAN, R. G. and J. M. KNOX: Treatment of Skin Cancer.
12 LYNCH, H. T.: Hereditary Factors in Carcinoma.
13 Tumours in Children, 2nd Edition. Edited by H. B. MARSDEN and J. K. STEWARD.
14 ODARTCHENKO, N.: Production Cellulaire Erythropoïétique.
15 SOKOLOFF, B.: Carcinoid and Serotonin.
16 JACOBS, M. L.: Malignant Lymphomas and Their Management.
17 Normal and Malignant Cell Growth. Edited by R. J. M. FRY, M. L. GRIEM, and W. H. KIRSTEN (Symposium).
18 ANGLESIO, E.: The Treatment of Hodgkin's Disease.
19 BANNASCH, P.: The Cytoplasm of Hepatocytes during Carcinogenesis. Electron- and Lightmicroscopical Investigations of the Nitrosomorpholineintoxicated Rat Liver.
20 Rubidomycin. A new Agent against Cancer. Edited by J. BERNARD, R. PAUL, M. BOIRON, C. JACQUILLAT, and R. MARAL.
21 Scientific Basis of Cancer Chemotherapy. Edited by G. MATHÉ (Symposium).
22 KOLDOVSKÝ, P.: Tumor Specific Transplantation Antigen.
23 FUCHS, W. A., J. W. Davidson, and H. W. FISCHER: Lymphography in Cancer. With contributions by G. JANTET and H. RÖSLER.
24 HAYWARD, J.: Hormones und Human Breast Cancer. An Account of 15 Years Study.
25 ROY-BURMAN, P.: Analogues of Nucleic Acid Components. Mechanisms of Action.
26 Tumors of the Liver. Edited by G. T. PACK and A. H. ISLAMI.
27 SZYMENDERA, J.: Bone Mineral Metabolism in Cancer.
28 MEEK, E. S.: Antitumour and Antiviral Substances of Natural Origin.
29 Aseptic Environments and Cancer Treatment. Edited by G. MATHÉ (Symposium).
30 Advances in the Treatment of Acute (Blastic) Leukemias. Edited by G. MATHÉ (Symposium).
31 DENOIX, P.: Treatment of Malignant Breast Tumors. Indications and Results.
32 NELSON, R. S.: Endoscopy in Gastric Cancer.
33 Experimental and Clinical Effects of L-Asparaginase. Edited by E. GRUNDMANN and H. F. OETTGEN (Symposium).
34 Chemistry and Biological Actions of 4-Nitroquinolin 1-Oxide. Edited by H. ENDO, T. ONO, and T. SUGIMURA.
35 PENN, I.: Malignant Tumors in Organ Transplant Recipients.
36 Current Concepts in the Management of Lymphoma and Leukemia. Edited by J. E. ULTMANN, M. L. GRIEM, W. H. KIRSTEN, and R. W. WISSLER (Symposium).
37 CHIAPPA, S., R. MUSUMECI, and C. USLENGHI: Endolymphatic Radiotherapy in Malignant Lymphomas. With contributions by G. BONADONNA, B. DAMASCELLI, G. FAVA, F. PIZZETTI, U. VERONESI.
38 KOLLER, P. C.: The Role of Chromosomes in Cancer Biology.
39 Current Problems in the Epidemiology of Cancer and Lymphomas. Edited by E. GRUNDMANN and H. TULINIUS (Symposium).
40 LANGLEY, F. A. and A. C. CROMPTON: Epithelial Abnormalities of the Cervix Uteri.
41 Tumours in a Tropical Country. A Survey of Uganda (1964–1968). Edited by A. C. TEMPLETON.
42 Breast Cancer: A Challenging Problem. Edited by M. L. GRIEM, E. V. JENSEN, J. E. ULTMANN, and R. W. WISSLER (Symposium).
43 Nomenclature, Methodology and Results of Clinical Trials in Acute Leukemias. Edited by G. MATHÉ, P. POUILLART, L. SCHWARZENBERG (Symposium).
44 Special Topics in Carcinogenesis. Edited by E. GRUNDMANN (Symposium).
45 KOLDOVSKÝ, P.: Carcinoembryonic Antigens.
46 Diagnosis and Therapy of Malignant Lymphoma. Edited by K. MUSSHOFF (Symposium).
47 Investigation and Stimulation of Immunity in Cancer Patients. Edited by G. MATHÉ and R. WEINER (Symposium).
48 Platinum Coordination Complexes in Cancer Chemotherapy. Edited by T. A. CONNORS and J. J. ROBERTS (Symposium).
49 Complications of Cancer Chemotherapy. Edited by G. MATHÉ and R. K. OLDHAM (Symposium).
50 Cancer Registry, Edited by E. GRUNDMANN and E. PEDERSEN (Symposium).

51 Gliomas. Current Concepts in Biology, Diagnosis and Therapy. Edited by J. HEKMATPANAH (Symposium).

52 The Ambivalence of Cytostatic Therapy. Edited by E. GRUNDMANN and R. GROSS (Symposium).

53 A. CLARYSSE, Y. KENIS, and G. MATHÉ: Cancer Chemotherapy.

54 Malignant Bone Tumors. Edited by E. GRUNDMANN.

55 MATHÉ, G.: Cancer Active Immunotherapy, Immunoprophylaxis, and Immunorestoration.

56 Lymphocytes, Macrophages, and Cancer. Edited by G. MATHÉ, I. FLORENTIN, and M.-C. SIMMLER (Symposium).

57 Breast Cancer: A Multidisciplinary Approach. Edited by G. ST. ARNEAULT, P. BAND, and L. ISRAËL (Symposium).

58 B. S. SCHOENBERG: Multiple Primary Malignant Neoplasms.

59 Selective Heat Sensitivity of Cancer Cells. Edited by A. ROSSI-FANELLI, R. CAVALIERE, B. MONDOVI, and G. MORICCA.

60 Tumors of the Male Genital System. Edited by E. GRUNDMANN and W. VAHLENSIECK (Symposium).

61 D. METCALF: Hemopoietic Colonies.

62 Tactics and Strategy in Cancer Treatment. Edited by G. MATHÉ (Symposium).

63 Antitumor Antibiotics. Edited by S. K. CARTER, H. UMEZAWA, J. DOUROS, and Y. SAKURAI (Symposium).

64 Lymphoid Neoplasias I: Classification, Categorization, Natural History.

65 Lymphoid Neoplasias II: Clinical and Therapeutic Aspects.
Lymphoid Neoplasias I & II. Proceedings of the 1977 CNRS-EORTC International Colloquium. Editors: G. MATHÉ, M. SELIGMANN, M. TUBIANA. Devided into two volumes.

66 Carcinogenic Hormones. Edited by C. H. LINGEMAN.

67/68 Adjuvant Therapies and Markers of Post-Surgical Minimal Residual Disease I & II. Proceedings of the 1978 Annual Plenary Meeting of the EORTC. Editors: G. BONADONNA, G. MATHÉ, S. E. SALMON. Divided into two volumes:

67 Markers and General Problems of Cancer Adjuvant Therapies.

68 Adjuvant Therapies of the Various Primary Tumors.

69 Strategies in Clinical Hematology. Edited by R. GROSS and K.-P. HELLRIEGEL.

70 New Anticancer Drugs. Edited by S. K. CARTER

71 Endocrine Treatment of Breast Cancer. Edited by B. HENNINGSEN, F. LINDER, C. STREICHELE.

72 CAWLEY, J. C., BURNS, G. F., HAYHOE, F. G. J.: Hairy-Cell Leukaemia

www.ingramcontent.com/pod-product-compliance
Lightning Source LLC
Chambersburg PA
CBHW061218240926
51846CB00006B/1272
* 9 7 8 3 6 4 2 8 1 4 3 9 6 *